MADE TO MEASURE

IMPROVE YOUR HEALTH BY FOCUSSING ON
WHAT MATTERS

DR. JESSE D. CARRIE, PH.D.

For my family,
for their support on my journey

TABLE OF CONTENTS

INTRODUCTION

"If I have seen farther than others, it is by standing on the shoulders of giants."

— ISAAC NEWTON

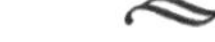

Why Should You Read This Book?

The opening quote is marvellous for two reasons: (1) it demonstrates a virtuous cycle that allows for continual expansion of the good things in life such as health; (2) it demonstrates humility and a sense of interconnection with all that have come before us. I would not be where I am today without all of the giants who have come before me. The knowledge gained from those who came before; the support of all, however near or far; and the blessings of being alive at this time have allowed for me to be where and who I am. I would like to return the favour; pay it forward.

Whenever we want (or need) to learn something that will benefit us, we should seek out a guide who has demonstrated experience in what we want to achieve. It is my goal to help serve as this guide for you- to enable you to see farther and achieve the life you want.

Who Am I, Anyway?

I've always had a love of food. I've been in the kitchen cooking since I was a teenager, in large part because I've always had a ravenous appetite, and I couldn't rely on my parents to *always* be in the kitchen making me something to eat. While I've never been the biggest guy in the room, I certainly ate that way (I was even nicknamed "tapeworm" during my hockey playing days). There were more than a few occasions where I might've eaten half my body weight in a day. (I'm not a big guy, so it's not **that** much...) Needless to say, my parents were relieved when I left for university, as their grocery bill plummeted.

Necessity is the mother of invention.

— PLATO

While at university, in part to living in a city renowned for its magnificent cuisine (Montréal) and in part to being a cash-strapped student, I came upon the mother of invention: necessity. I had to feed myself, cheaply, and with all of the wonderful options available, I was able to test out a lot of different cuisines. During this period, I also went from a near carnivore to vegetarian, but more on the reasons why shortly. (**Spoiler alert:** It was NOT to impress a girl, shocking as that may sound.)

While I ate immense amounts of food, I also developed

certain allergies along the way. Around 17 or 18 years of age, I developed an allergy to cow's milk. (About half of the allergies you have are developed as an adult.) Previously, I had been drinking several litres (at least half a gallon) a day. Yet at that time, my throat would close up whenever I drank milk. I had to make a decision: continue with the ability to swallow comfortably, or give up drinking milk. It was a tough call, but I finally went with the ability to swallow.

This was the start of my paying attention to what I ate and how it made me feel.

As I mentioned, I was a cash-strapped university student, and what's the ultimate nourishment for poor folk? Bread! I ate wheat in all of its delicious guises: bread, baguettes, croissants, noodles/pasta, pita, naan, pizza, and bagels. My newfound vegetarianism also meant that I was substituting the meat products I used to eat with the vegetarian version — "pepperoni", "chicken", you name it. All of these had wheat gluten in them for texture and protein.

By my mid-twenties, after most meals, my stomach would swell out like I was pregnant and I would need time to digest. I also needed at least 8.5 hours of sleep every night just to feel normal.

At this time, I had started to teach at the local university. One of the topics I covered was sanitation. I was explaining to my mostly very sheltered students how great it is to have indoor plumbing and sewers. We also did some fun math about how much water use is required for this great service. It quickly became evident that I was using the facilities a bit more frequently than most. My wife did not need anyone to tell her this, especially as our house at that time only had one bathroom. (My wife is a saint.)

My wife kindly suggested that I try giving up gluten, as I had pretty much all of the symptoms for Celiac disease. I fought her on this for a while, because I LOVED everything gluten. Old habits die hard — my bread eating ways hadn't really changed since my university days. I mean, a perfectly prepared baguette or fresh baked bread? C'mon! So tasty.

I finally decided to listen to reason. (Yes, this is admitting my wife was right... again.) I decided to eliminate gluten from my diet for a few days to see how I would feel. I was VERY sceptical this would relieve my symptoms. Lo and behold, it was like a switch got turned on. I felt better the next day. I realise this is unusual, but bear with me.

Prior to this point, while I pretty much never got colds or flus, I would get struck with just about anything gut-related. Now I'm virtually ironclad everywhere. It's great. I also need less sleep to function normally, don't spend an hour or so on the couch after a meal (I can actually do stuff in the evening now) and let's just say my wife doesn't need to be as saintly any more.

This change was the frying-pan-to-the-face hit I needed to realise that we really need to pay attention to what we put into our bodies and how this makes us feel. To be clear, I am not advocating that everyone adopt a dairy-free, gluten-free diet. This has helped me immensely, but you need to listen to your body and see what is and isn't working for you. This book will help guide you on how to make some of these decisions by showing the science behind nutrition.

Ain't Nuthin' but a G(eek) Thang

I've also had a lifelong love of figuring things out. I love looking for patterns and taking things apart (and rebuilding them). Part of this is understanding the chemical building blocks of everything we know — food, materials, and the environment around us. I even have a periodic table of the elements shower curtain.

(There are, apparently, limits to how much a spouse will condone. This may only be used in the basement bathroom.) Yep, I'm a bit of a geek.

I've spent over two decades studying, researching and working in chemistry-related fields. Much of this time has been spent focusing on how to analyse all sorts of things, for all sorts of different chemical elements and compounds. I've analysed water, soil, rocks and minerals and countless biological species and foodstuffs as well as less common analyses like fossil fuels and nuclear materials. In short, I've pretty much done it all.

Throughout this time, I've worked with consulting firms, governmental health agencies, governmental natural resource agencies (including fisheries), the oil and gas industry as well as the nuclear industry. This work has taken me across the globe to four continents. I've seen the differences, but more importantly, I've seen the similarities that unite us all. This broad experience has also allowed me to see patterns that likely would not have happened otherwise.

Simplicity on the Far Side of Complexity

"For the simplicity that lies this side of complexity, I would not give a fig, but for the simplicity that lies on the other side of complexity, I would give my life."

— Oliver Wendell Holmes

Put differently, a Zen mind is a beginner's mind. After learning, struggling with and experiencing a lot of things on a given topic, that topic then becomes simple and teachable to others.

When you combine a lifelong love of food and an intense desire to figure things out — *and the practical experience to back it up* — good things result. I can see patterns where others might struggle to. Once you can see the patterns in the complex, you start to see simplicity on the far side of complexity. Once you've got simplicity on the far side of complexity, you can start helping others. And that is what I want to do here.

So let's get going, alright?

PART I

MEASUREMENT AND UNCERTAINTY AND HOW THIS AFFECTS YOUR HEALTH

1
———

MEASUREMENT AND UNCERTAINTY

If you don't measure it, you can't improve it.

— Peter Drucker

Don't measure anything unless the data helps you make a better decision or change your actions.

— Seth Godin

WE LIVE in an age where information is so readily available that it literally makes our heads hurt. Not only that, but the sheer volume of information is made worse by conflicting accounts from a whole series of experts. Especially when it comes to your health.

You may be asking yourself: Should I eat fat? Should I eat carbohydrates (carbs)? If so, how much? How much protein do

I need to eat? What minerals and vitamins do I really need? What's with those food labels, and why is some information captured and not others? What the heck do these numbers even mean?!

The trouble is, we're all unique. Someone will find something that works for them — and probably many others — and shout it out from their soapbox. Take the ketogenic (high fat, low carb, moderate protein) diet. It works wonders for many people. Contrary to what many think, the high fat in this diet typically leads to a lot of fat loss. Yet it will not work for someone else, leading to energy crashes and sluggishness. What's up with that?

We often forget that there's no single, simple answer to solve our problems. There's nuance to every situation.

What's more is what most of us don't know, or aren't aware of: how things are actually measured, and what those measurements actually mean.

By measuring something, we focus our attention on it. By focussing our attention on something, we can take action to bring it into existence or improve upon what's already there. Sometimes it's simply an attempt to figure what's already there, which helps us determine a certain degree of "normal", like body temperature so we know whether or not we have a fever. From there, we can then know what to do in the event that things aren't "normal". Again with the body temperature example, if we're running hot, cooling the body down by whatever means is usually the tactic taken.

However, we need to know that what we're measuring is actually good. We need to know how accurate those measurements are, and plan accordingly. Different things have different degrees of accuracy associated with them.

Have you ever driven a car when the fuel gauge is showing empty? How empty is empty? Odds are you can still drive a fair distance before the car literally runs out of gas. Hopefully you can make it to a gas station before then!

Bakers will tell you that you need to measure things by weight, not volume, to get things just right. It's a bit more work, but as they say, the proof is in the pudding.

As for anything science-related, everything is exact, right? Scientists can measure time down to nanoseconds with atomic clocks and can tell you how far apart atoms are on the silicon microchips powering your smartphone. Same thing goes for those nutrition facts on food, right?

Umm... To be polite, you'd be a little off the mark with that last one.

ANYTHING THAT IS alive is complex. And anything that is complex has a range of possible configurations. To describe an entire class of something with one label is, well, not a good idea. We've been over this in many, many cases. We even have words to describe this: racism, sexism, ageism. Let's look at a concrete numerical example. Take height for example: we could state that the average man is 170 cm (5'8") tall. It doesn't take a genius to figure out that there are a lot of men shorter, and taller, than that. By pretty wide stretches in either direction, to boot.

What nutrition fact labels are telling us is that all men are 170 cm tall. That's it, that's all. Height has no impact on basketball players, right? Or racehorse jockeys?

Wait! Am I saying that nutrition fact labels are basically worthless?

No.

What I am saying is that there are ranges to any kind of measurement involving living things and that we need to understand the uncertainty, or fuzziness, in how these measurements are made.

We need to know how far from that average we need to go to include most of the possibilities as well as the odds of finding those possibilities in that range. Taking height again, if we now assume that virtually all men will be between 140 and 210 cm (4'8" and 6'8"), we can then apply that knowledge to a whole series of things: what size pants to make (at least in length), how big to make seats, how big to make doorways. Or how many people can be crammed into an airplane without complaining too much. (Clearly, this knowledge can also be used for evil.)

Of course, making pants and doorways is a lot simpler than optimising someone's nutrition.

Fuzzy Logic

The other side of measurement is the application of it, especially where actions need to be taken, like when you get test results from your doctor. Let's face it — if we don't take action from our measurements, there's no point in doing them in the first place.

As alluded to above, things are never clear cut. Let's look at an example where things get a little fuzzy.

Let's say a measurement has a 10% error rate (this is actually really common, and pretty good, too). So if we measure something between 100 and 1000, we would consider ourselves good analysts if we get anywhere between 90 and 110 on the low end and 900 and 1100 on the high end.

Now let's put this in a context of acceptable ranges that your doctor might tell you about. Again, let's assume the normal range is 100 to 1000. For anything below 100, you would be considered deficient and need some kind of supplementation. For anything above 1000, you would be considered to have excessive, and typically toxic, amounts of it, and need to find a way to cut back.

Now remember, there's a 10% error in the measurement. Let's say your test result comes back at 105, which puts you in the "normal" category. But it could be as low 94.5 (below the "normal" threshold, falling into the deficient zone) or as high as 115.5 if a few more measurements were made. Let's look at some visuals to help make sense of this:

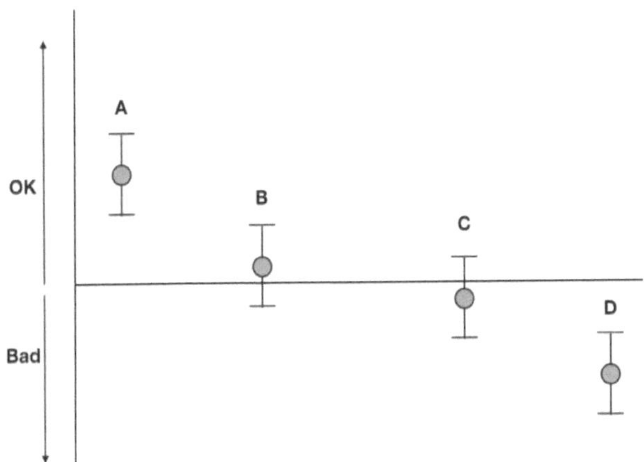

From here, it's pretty obvious that case A falls completely in the OK range. Similarly, it's obvious case D falls completely in the Bad range (for example, you would be deficient or, if we were to flip the image upside down, you would have toxic amounts of something). What's not so clear is what happens in cases B and C. Is B really in the OK zone, or might it be bad? Likewise, is C really bad, or might it be OK?

Let's look at some practical applications.

Let's say your initial test result falls in the "normal" range.

Your doctor tells you you have nothing to worry about. Yet you don't feel quite right, and still experience the symptoms that might occur with a deficiency. You might want to ask for a re-test, or what course of action might be taken if you were to have a deficiency.

The same idea goes on the other end of the scale (just flip the image above upside down to get a visual). You might have really high amounts of something, yet you feel just fine. In this case, you might *not* want to take a course of action, as the side effects might be worse than the condition itself.

So what do you do?

I honestly can't answer this for you. It is something you'll have to think about and discuss with your health care provider. Just know that things are often not black and white. Listen to your body. It will tell you if you're on the right track or not.

~

Information Overload

More information is better, right?

You could get all of your food analysed before you eat it. Obviously, this would lead to a lot of delays in actually getting your food. And increases in costs. While no company will admit this, laws requiring food be analysed before being marketed costs something; these costs WILL be passed on to the consumer. (Shameless plug: It's not all bad — the huge boom in the number of chemists needed to do these analyses provides a lot of job security to chemists like me.) More detailed analyses, such as finding out exactly what amino acids make up your protein could be done; you could also determine the exact fats making up the total fat content; ditto the sugar molecules in carbohydrates. This could be done by location and season. And that's just the macronutrients!

Phew! Too. Much. Information!

We are all well aware that we live in an age of information overload. Adding more information is clearly not going to be helpful, at least not without some way of filtering out the noise. Too much information simply leads to short-circuiting the brain and ultimately, inaction. Analysis paralysis. It's like looking at the sun: we all enjoy the light it provides, but if we look directly at it (in other words, collect WAY more "information"), we can't see a thing, and it usually takes a little while before we can see properly again. Which is probably why we like to order a pizza or something similar after a long day at work. Our brains are usually fried by the end of the day, and thinking about what to make for supper often becomes too hard a task.

My point is that we could spend all of our time measuring things to the smallest detail in the hopes of making the best choices for ourselves. Taken to the extreme, it's not only missing the forest for the trees, but missing the trees themselves for the leaves.

There are costs associated with collecting all of this information. For one, your money is important. You want to have the best health possible, without breaking the bank. Similarly, your time is very valuable. (I would argue more valuable than your money.) Do you want to spend hours upon hours every week ensuring that you've measured everything you need exactly so, or do you want to spend that time doing stuff you enjoy? Perhaps hanging out at the beach, enjoying a nice evening with friends and family or getting out and enjoying the natural beauty near you or on a trip?

Throwing the Baby Out With the Bathwater

Another important thing to do is not throw the baby out with the bathwater. Keeping a critical eye on research and reports can help weed out good (or bad) information.

So what do I mean by this?

Science basically works according to this paradigm:

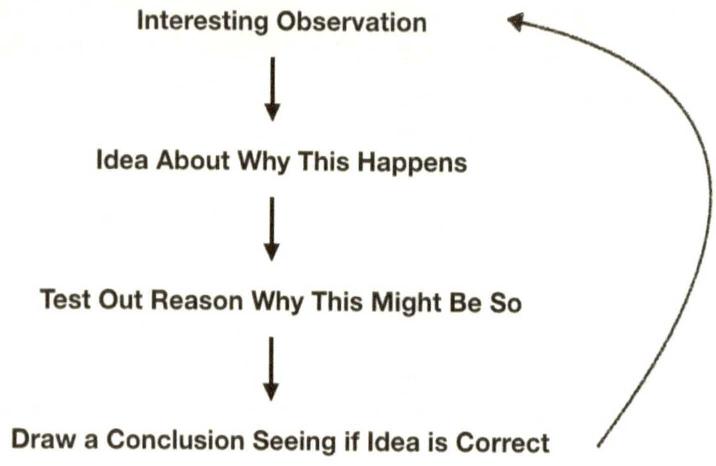

HUMANS HAVE ACTUALLY DONE this for as long as we've been a species. A quick example: Let's look at one of our caveman ancestors. For the sake of our story, let's call him Dave. Caveman Dave is hungry, and notices that, for a few weeks each year, this one plant produces a nice red fruit (*observation*). Maybe I can eat this fruit, thinks Dave (*idea, or hypothesis*). To see if he can, Dave eats one of these fruits one day (*test idea*). Hunger is satisfied; Dave does not keel over in pain. Conclusion: eat fruit = less hunger = no pain = good idea to eat more fruit.

Most of the time, this works well. The trouble with this is that sometimes a pattern is found in a certain group that might not actually be there, or isn't applicable outside of the group studied.

Looking at Dave again and, based on his earlier success with eating red fruit, he would probably try to eat another red fruit. Again, success! Lucky Dave.

After a string of successes, Dave now thinks that all red fruit are good. While out exploring, he uses his knowledge of red fruit = good and gorges on a bunch of red fruit. This time, things don't go so well. Dave is in considerable pain, doubled over. To make matters worse, he's out hunting alone, and those sabre-toothed tigers aren't extinct yet. Ouch.

This is a classic case of correlation (red fruit = good) is not causation (while many red fruit are good, some are toxic).

The correlation-causation problem can manifest itself in a number of ways:

- (1) When an observed pattern is linked to a specific outcome (this is the correlation). However, sometimes things just *happen* to be linked to certain outcomes. Probably the worst offender of this is Ansel Keys, who believed fat intake was causing people to become fat, which led to decades of blind faith in fat-free diets and a witch hunt on all things fat, which we finally seem to be freeing ourselves of little by little. (If you eat a lot of fat, especially when coupled with more than adequate amounts of carbs and protein, you most definitely will get fat.)
- (2) Extrapolation beyond the given population in a dataset. This may shock you, but well-off white guys tend to have different health outcomes than subsistence farmers in a desert. This one is also deadly, and the reason why there's so much bad advice out there, or more appropriately, why a lot of advice **simply doesn't work for you.**

For example, some people can tolerate dairy well (mainly of northern European and northeast African descent), while much of the global population has varying degrees of lactose intolerance. So the edicts to avoid all dairy products might not necessarily apply to you, although the odds are good that they do. (Personally, dairy and I don't get along too well, so I avoid it most of the time.)

Another interesting bit is the omega-3 fats. The original impetus for studying these fats is the Inuit. Inuit survived on basically nothing but fat and protein from marine animals (seals, whales, and to a lesser extent, fish and polar bears). While eating all of this fat, they have virtually no heart disease or strokes (the story is completely different now that many have adopted a typical Western diet). But what's interesting is that they have adapted genetically to this source of food. They are able to metabolise these fats in a healthy way, while the same doesn't appear to hold up as well in most of the rest of the world. This is not to say that you shouldn't be eating omega-3s. You should. They're an essential fat, meaning your body can't make them. The point is that you don't need to load up on them as your main source of fat.

So why do we have this correlation-causation problem in the first place?

There is a reason for this: testing out several unknowns at once is really hard. Do you remember trying to solve those math problems in school where you had more than one unknown? It either required a lot more work, or was impossible (literally).

The reason why science only does one thing at a time, besides the basic tenet of science to examine one thing at a time, is that it's really difficult to get money to study many things at once and it's also really hard to determine effects from multiple things acting together. New algorithms and advanced computing have only been able to help tease things out for the past decade or two, and even then, very few in any field are proficient in this.

All this to say, scientists really are doing the best they can to figure things out. It takes time, and sometimes new information comes along that contradicts the earlier stuff, or perhaps more appropriately, boundaries are drawn as to where the data actually applies.

There's obviously a lot of information out there, and given that some things work for some people and not for others, you really need to become your own advocate. One constant is to eat lots of veggies, and to mix and match as much as possible. When you go grocery shopping, try a new vegetable and then look up some recipes that might appeal to you. Who knows? You might discover your new favourite food.

Another thing to keep in mind is scale. So many reports will indicate that something that's not good for us has been detected in some kind of food, water, or our bodies. For example, I can pretty much guarantee that you have some Teflon in you, and not the metaphorical kind that allows stuff to roll right off of you. Even if you don't use Teflon-coated (most non-stick) pans. Conversely, you might hear or read that something *good* has been detected in something — like omega-3 fatty acids in certain oils. Yet you will almost never hear *how much*. This "*how much*" is really important.

Sometimes what we actually measure is less than one in a trillion (that's 11 zeroes after the decimal). More often than not, this is a testament to how good we've become at detecting things — not something to be overly worried about. Other times, much less is present than is required for a relevant dose (looking at you, omega-3 eggs!). The flip side is that, depending upon regulations, nutrition labels can state something like "zero trans fats" when the unit being measured is much less than what you'll actually eat. Because we all know that you'll only eat 5 chips at once, right? (Serving size is pretty sketchy.)

These last two cases are particularly bad examples of marketing being used against us, and will usually fool us into thinking something is better for us than it is.

On the other hand, sometimes we get so caught up in something that can be good, that we go overboard and end up consuming enough to make us sick. Maybe not immediately, but definitely within a shorter timeframe than we expect. This is especially true with supplements that concentrate certain nutrients. At some point or another, your body will tell you that you've had too much of a good thing. For example, you definitely need protein, but if you get too much, you'll wear your kidneys out in short order. Not exactly something you want to do.

We're all familiar with the story of Goldilocks and the Three Bears. But finding that *just right* amount can be really hard, especially when different things have different amounts of "just rightness".

In the chapters that follow, I'll show you how to make the best choices with regards to your nutrition so that you can use those precious resources (your time and money) for what you want most. I'll describe how things like fat, fibre and minerals are analysed and how to find the best way to get those nutrients. Sometimes what is measured isn't even what it's supposed to be. Other times, there's way less than what is measured. Sometimes there's a lot more.

As you might have guessed, this book is not a one-size-fits-all approach. You are unique. You need to eat that way, too!

PART II

THE BIG PICTURE: MACRONUTRIENTS

2
___

FAT: FRIEND OR (DELICIOUS) FOE?

The function of education is to teach one to think intensively and to think critically.

— MARTIN LUTHER KING, JR.

Hey, Fathead!

Hold on! Why am I starting a chapter on fat with a quote to use your noggin by Martin Luther King? And isn't calling someone a fathead pretty much the opposite of that quote?

Actually, we're all fatheads. Our brains are composed predominantly of fat (about 60% or so). If we had to pick one organ to prize above all others, it would probably be our brains. They allow us to think, control our bodies and be creative. And this all requires fat. Hence, we're all fatheads.

So why do I insist on calling all of us fatheads? What's really behind this?

The best way to think of the brain is as a really complex, interconnected electrical circuit. It's like your house's electrical system on steroids... on steroids (... on steroids). As with the electricity you're likely familiar with, for proper transmission, the electrical cables have to be insulated. If not, the electrical charge will connect to whatever's next to it, and the charge won't get passed on to its intended destination. If you've ever accidentally touched a live wire, you know this is not a good thing. Ouch! In your house, car or electronics, these cables are insulated in some type of plastic. Plastics are basically fat. Chemically, they're very similar, and do a similar thing: they don't conduct electricity.

Your nerves and neurons are very similar. They have an insulating layer (known as myelin) with the conducting "cable" on the inside. Myelin is predominantly fat. It ensures that the signal gets to pass from one spot in the body to another. This is NOT something you want short-circuiting.

Now for your brain: it is *loaded* with neurons, which means lots of myelin, and thus, lots of fat.

This is probably THE MOST important reason for eating good fat in your diet. By good fat, I mean two things: (1) not the trans (aka hydrogenated) fats we keep hearing are bad for us; and (2) not rancid fat. Rancid fat comes from unsaturated fats (yes, those fats that are typically considered very healthy!) that have been exposed to oxygen to form dangerous peroxides (reactive oxygen species, or ROS) that cause a chain reaction of negative effects in the body. Fortunately, our noses and taste buds can tell us right away if a fat is rancid — no matter the source, they all smell more or less the same, and taste pretty gross.

Another way to look at this is to NOT eat a low-fat diet. I'm not saying eat nothing but fat, but I am saying you'll need to eat a pretty decent amount of fat to optimise your brain health.

We'll cover what kinds of fats a little later. And no, eating fat does not make you fat, provided you don't eat way more than you need.

Your body can make some fat, but not all that you need. It's why you have arms, hands, legs and feet — you can go get the nutrition you need from your environment. We are, after all, not plants. (They don't move, so they need to produce everything they need themselves.)

By going out and getting your fat, you save your body a lot of work, allowing for better things to work. This is like buying your clothes from a store instead of harvesting the materials to make the fibres, spinning them into usable fibres, then actually making your clothes. By buying your clothes already made, you free up your time and abilities for other tasks. Same thing for your body.

So what happens if you don't get enough of the good fat to sustain your brain? Let's go back to the electrical wire analogy. If you don't have enough fat, then your nerves and neurons will start to have gaps in their coverage, so to speak. Systems start to short out, as the signals don't reach their proper destinations.

Remember the telephone game you played as a kid? The message reaching the end was pretty much never the same as that at the start because the signal got mixed up along the way. Mixed messages rarely lead to anything good. Heck, you might even be reading this book because of the mixed messages you keep hearing about food!

As the brain starts to lose its proper connections, brain fog can start to set in, leading eventually to things like dementia and Alzheimer's. For any of you who have experienced this with loved ones, you know it's a scary way to finish up your life. It's definitely something none of us want to experience.

So remember — being a fathead is a good thing. Make sure you eat some good fats to keep your brain (and body) healthy.

Good sources are from plants (olives, avocados, nuts and seeds such as hemp, flax and chia) as well as aquatic sources (seaweed, fish and the like).

One precautionary note about marine sources: chemical contaminants tend to accumulate in the bodies of larger and older fish. If you're buying supplements of fish oil (or omega-3 oils), know that it's generally better to have fats sourced from fish low on the food chain (for example, sardines and roe, or fish eggs). The same thing goes for eating whole fish — smaller fish will be lower in contaminants.

Or go to the foundation — algae. For those wishing to not eat fish, it is possible to eat the algae that feed most of the aquatic food web. Like us, most fish get their fats from their diets and don't actually make them themselves, so this way, you're going right to the source. By eating the algae, you're also drastically reducing the amount of contaminants you'll be consuming, plus they generally have a lot of important micronutrients in them as well. Remember — algae are the plants of the sea, so they need to make everything themselves.

A word of caution: algae are, to be polite, an acquired taste (I'm looking at you, spirulina and chlorella!). If you're able to eat it directly, you're a stronger person than I am (and most people I know). On the bright side, most suppliers have caught on to this and now offer spirulina and chlorella in gel caps, so unless you bite into it before swallowing, it should make its way into your system without offending your taste buds. Win-win!

All animals are created equal, but some are more equal than others.

— GEORGE ORWELL, FROM ANIMAL FARM

FATS SHARE a certain likeness to that section of George Orwell's *Animal Farm* where the pigs set out some ground rules. They are generally considered to always give nine calories per gram (not entirely true, as we'll see shortly), yet they behave very differently in the body.

By now, you've heard of saturated and unsaturated fats. You might have even heard of medium chain fats, which by default would lead you to believe, correctly, that there are small (short) and large (long) chains as well. Let's take a look at them.

So what's the difference between these short-chain fatty acids you might be hearing about and the long-chain ones?

Fatty acids are basically made up of two parts: (1) the fatty tail, and (2) the polar, or water-soluble head (the "acid"). You can kind of think of them like this:

Carbon atoms ("fatty")

O

OH

Acid ("carboxyl")

Because it's a lot easier to draw a squiggly line than write letters, scientists tend to draw fats as squiggly lines. That's right — like everyone else, scientists like to make their life easier whenever they can. Fats generally have an even number of carbon atoms in their structure, as this is how they're made (two carbons at a time). So you'll see fats with 6, 8, 10, 12, 14, 16, 18 up to about 26 carbon atoms (normally named C_6, C_8, C_{12}, etc.). One thing to keep in mind is that as the fatty part gets longer, the molecule becomes more and more solid, and less and less water soluble. For example, the C_2 fatty acid, acetic acid (aka vinegar) is very water soluble and liquid at room temperature. Yet C_{10} (a medium-chain fat; one of the main fats in coconut oil) is solid at room temperature (but melts around 25°C/77°F) and C_{18} (stearic acid) is definitely solid (one of the fats found in butter).

There is a catch — unsaturated fats (meaning they're short a few hydrogen atoms) stay liquid at much lower temperatures than their saturated counterparts. This is in part why fish, particularly coldwater fish like salmon, have higher amounts of unsaturated fat— they'd stiffen up otherwise. And it's why they're such a great source of unsaturated fats.

Another quick note about saturated fats and unsaturated fats: virtually all of the short- and medium-chain fats are saturated, yet are extremely healthy to eat. So it really comes down to knowing what kind of fat is saturated that you're eating — the longer the chain (particularly past about C_{20}), the harder it is for your body to make good use of it.

As mentioned above, unsaturated fats mean that there are at least two hydrogen atoms "missing" from a fully saturated carbon-carbon link (carbon can have up to four bonds with other atoms). What this does is create a bit of rigidity to the fat structure. Remember the squiggly lines above? Those squiggly lines can move in just about any direction, so if need be, the fat molecule can bend or straighten out depending on its environment. Those unsaturated fats? Not so lucky.

There are two types of unsaturation: cis and trans. Now we've all heard of trans fats, and that they're bad. But why? Believe it or not, trans fats are actually a lot more stable than cis fats. Before we really understood the biology of unsaturated fats, it was thought to be a great idea to reduce the amount of rancidity in fats, which would allow for food to last much longer. And it does indeed last longer. Crisco, anyone?

You may have noticed that coconut oil tends to come in clear containers, while other vegetable oils like olive oil come in green- or amber-coloured containers. This is because olive oil, which is loaded with unsaturated fats, is particularly prone to becoming rancid, and light (both visible and UV) speeds up the process. By having a coloured container, this slows down the rate at which the oil becomes rancid. Since coconut oil is almost all saturated fat, it's much less prone to developing off-flavours.

(**NERD ALERT**: Rancidity happens when oxygen (such as in air) reacts with the unsaturated fat to form a peroxide. Nasty, nasty stuff that is. Peroxides react dangerously with just about everything — they're the worst of the "free radicals", and the main reason behind the advice to get enough antioxidants. If you've ever cleaned a wound with hydrogen peroxide and felt the sting, that's the peroxide reacting with everything you put it on. I'm pretty sure you wouldn't dream of eating hydrogen peroxide, but that's basically what's happening on a smaller scale when you eat rancid fat.)

FYI, hydrogenated vegetable oil is another way to say trans fats. Fortunately, although the evidence has long been established, the US and Canada have finally made trans fats illegal (in June 2018 and September 2018, respectively). Hallelujah!

Short End of the Stick

There's increasing evidence that short-chain fatty acids can help reduce inflammation, reduce insulin resistance and help with brain health.

Short-chain fatty acids are generally considered to just be from one to five carbon atoms. You may be familiar with a two-carbon fatty acid: vinegar. Seriously — acetic acid is vinegar. Short-chain fatty acids (SCFA) are also made by gut bacteria and have a whole suite of health effects (generally good ones — mainly related to reduced inflammation in the gut, reducing insulin resistance). The ketogenic diet is reliant upon these for fuels — the fuel that is used is typically C_3 and C_4 acids (propionic and butyric acids, respectively), and will often come partly oxidised (this is the "keto" part, which is short for "ketone"). Exercise also helps your gut bacteria make more of these SCFA.

Another great source of SCFA? Fermented foods. Sauerkraut (made the old-fashioned way), kimchi and kefir are some of the more popular fermented foods. If you're feeling adventurous, you can ferment all sorts of things — all you need is water, salt and some containers that can be sealed.

The next bunch is the medium-chain fatty acids. They're all the rage these days, though they sometimes go by the moniker "MCT" (Medium-Chain Triglycerides, where triglycerides are another word for fat). For the most part, the most important source of MCT are coconuts. Coconut oil is primarily C_8 to C_{12} fatty acids. There's increasing research that these compounds are great for the brain, as their structure allows them to pass through the blood-brain barrier.

So we've covered small and medium... on to large!

This would typically be what you would consider "fat". These range from C_{14} to about C_{22}, although larger fats exist (docosohexaenoic acid, or DHA, is C_{26} and is involved in a lot of brain stuff). It's really here that the difference between saturated and unsaturated fats becomes prevalent. Generally speaking, fats from plants will contain a much higher proportion of unsaturated fats (either mono- or polyunsaturated; the difference is the number of unsaturated bonds — mono for one unsaturated bond, poly for more than one).

It's also here that the difference between saturated and unsaturated becomes important. Unsaturated fats come in two flavours: (1) the more stable trans form (yes, *those* trans fats); and (2) the less stable, but biologically important cis form. Unsaturated fats are almost always in the cis form (think of a clothespin):

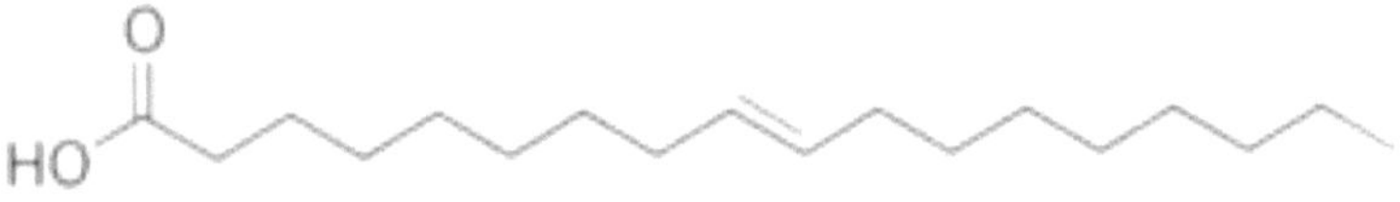

trans-Oleic acid

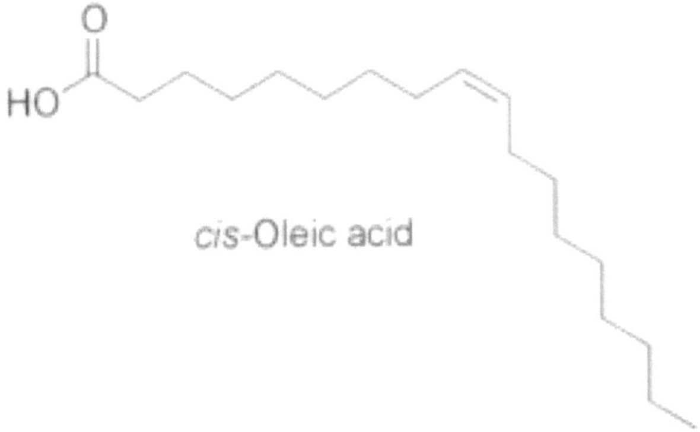

cis-Oleic acid

When you add more than one unsaturated bond (polyunsaturated fats), this allows the fat to fold into tighter spaces and to coil up, which is what happens with polyunsaturated fats. However, this feature also makes them more prone to oxidation. In other words, they're more likely to form reactive oxygen species and becoming rancid.

From the Alpha to the Omega

Omega-3 fatty acid simply means that the first unsaturated bond is at the third carbon from the end of the fatty tail. Omega-6 means it's the sixth carbon from the end. (The use of "omega" simply means "from the end", as omega is the last letter of the Greek alphabet.) Omega-3s are generally considered anti-inflammatory and generally amazing for your health, while omega-6s are often considered inflammatory. The latter are mostly found in corn, canola and other vegetable oils and used in most processed foods, which is in part why they get such a bad rap.

With all of the recent push to eat unsaturated fat and avoid saturated fat, you need to be mindful of what's actually going on. Most of the earlier science based on saturated fat being the scourge of the human race is actually mistaken — it doesn't make you fat (per se), nor does it plug you up and make you ripe for a heart attack or stroke.

As mentioned above, unsaturated fat certainly has its benefits, but you have to make sure you're getting it fresh — it becomes rancid really easily, and this rancidity can be deadly. Give any sensitive oils such as olive or nut oils a good sniff test before eating them. Your nose knows — if it smells a little off, just pitch it.

Egg on Your Face

You were probably told that cholesterol is bad for you, or at least to limit the amount you eat to avoid any heart health issues. Yet cholesterol is needed for most of your endocrine system (hormones, etc.). You need it. Big time.

Did you know that cholesterol is also needed to make Vitamin D? (Vitamin D is actually a hormone, not a nutrient, but old names tend to stick around.) You might know that Vitamin D is required for good bone health, which is why it's recommended to have it with calcium. In fact, you probably either take it as a supplement (straight up or part of a multivitamin) or if you consume dairy, you're getting a dose of it, because it's added to all milk and yogurt.

So if you like things like strong bones, a robust immune system and flashing those pearly whites, you're gonna want to make sure you eat at least some cholesterol.

This is great news if you thought those egg-white omelettes

needed a little something. You can eat those whole-egg ones without worry.

3
___

CARBOHYDRATES: SO SIMPLE, IT'S COMPLEX

Everything is energy and that's all there is to it.

— ALBERT EINSTEIN

∿

Fact can be stranger than fiction. There is indeed a Professor Popsicle (no relation to Popsicle Pete, purveyor of sugary frozen treats). Of course, that's not his real name — it's Gordon Giesbrecht, and he's a professor at the University of Manitoba in Winnipeg, Canada. For the uninitiated, Winnipeg has a reputation, even among Canadians, as a bitterly cold place where winter persists 8 months of the year. It frequently hits -40°C (-40°F) in the winter, with daytime highs around -20°C (-4°F) or colder on a regular basis for most of January and February. Because it's on the prairies, there aren't any hills or many trees to block the wind, so it's also windy most of the time, which makes it feel even colder. So yeah, it can get cold. (I lived there for 10 years. It's actually really nice, even in the winter.)

Anyway, what's so different about Professor Popsicle is that he studies hypothermia (when the body gets too cold to function), and intentionally lets himself get hypothermic (he's been on the David Letterman show a few times immersing himself in ice baths; google the videos if you're curious). So he knows a thing or two about how to get out of hypothermia and get warm again.

Besides the obvious of removing yourself from whatever is freezing you, would you believe that it's actually better to drink a cold sugary drink than a glass of warm water? What's up with that?

As it turns out, the body gets warmer from the sugar boost because it has to metabolise it, and this generates energy, which in turn leads to heat. Warm water will help some, but not as much as the energy boost. As most of you are aware, sugars fall into the carbohydrate group on nutrition labels.

CARBOHYDRATES, or carbs for short, are necessary ingredients for life. The name comes from a simplification of the atomic composition of a sugar molecule: Carbo (1 carbon atom, or "C") and hydrate (water, or H_2O) for an overall $C\,H_2O$, although in reality it's closer to $C_6H_{12}O_6$ for a single sugar molecule. And that's the simplified version.

You can kind of think of the different sugars like a Mr. Potato Head. There's the general potato and a bunch of holes to insert the different appendages (eyes, nose, mouth, arms, etc.). There really isn't anything stopping you from putting an arm in an eye socket or vice versa. The neat thing here, like when playing with a Mr. Potato Head, is that within a given set, you can more or less mix and match to create different versions of Mr. Potato Head, or in life, carbohydrates. Just a few of them look like this:

Glucose

Fructose

Sucrose

YOU HAVE the monosaccharides (simple sugars like glucose and fructose), the disaccharides (like sucrose, made up of one glucose and one fructose), and beyond that, the polysaccharides (things like starch, or cellulose).

Carbs come in either the six-member rings (pyranoses, like glucose and galactose) or the five-member rings (furanoses, like fructose and ribose). Glucose and galactose (simple sugars) have the same overall structure (6-member ring, or hexagon), except that at one point, an oxygen bond goes in one direction (say, "up"), while in the other, it goes in the opposite while still being connected to the same carbon atom. You can kind of think of this like having your right arm in your right arm socket, but in one case, it's how you would normally see it, while in the other, instead of defaulting to the hanging down position, it's always up. Overall, it's the same connection, but you can imagine that the function will be different. Same thing applies with the sugar molecules.

You probably won't notice much of a difference putting the eyes in upside down or the left arm in the right arm socket and vice versa, but those subtle differences will have an effect. Either a different type of bacteria will be able to use it more readily (and then become more prevalent in your gut), or it will act like a different kind of key into the "locks" present in many bodily sensors.

DNA

We've all heard of DNA. It stands for DeoxyriboNucleic Acid. The "D" part, *deoxyribo*, refers to the fact that a component of DNA is ribose ("ribo"), a sugar, that is missing an oxygen atom ("de-oxy"). So you obviously need ribose to live.

Ribose and fructose are the two most important 5-ring sugars. What's interesting however, is that your body treats them totally different than 6-ring sugars, such as glucose and galactose. 5-ring sugars go first to the liver to be transformed, often as fat. (Scientists know this because they can label compounds radiologically, normally through C-14, carbon's radioactive isotope, and follow them throughout the body.) This is why a lot of people are saying to avoid eating fruit if you want to lose weight. The trouble with this is that fruit is more than just fructose. But that's a topic for another chapter.

The other main sugars, glucose and galactose, are used up as energy sources during one of the body's main two metabolic pathways (the citric acid cycle). It's these sugars that are measured in the blood when "blood sugar" is being measured, and give us the glycemic index that diabetics are well acquainted with. It's also how to cheat at the glycemic index, as fructose doesn't really count in that index, yet obviously has numerous health repercussions.

What's important to note is that unless you're using up the sugar immediately, it's more than likely going to be transformed into fat for storage for later use. The body primarily transforms sugar into palmitic acid (a 16-carbon fat). Palmitic acid, a saturated fat, has been shown to be involved in certain cancers and heart disease. (Remember that useful nugget about "correlation is not causation"?)

The trouble is, to transform sugar into fat, you need to do a lot of work — the sugar must be "reduced" into a fat. This means that all of the oxygen atoms present in sugar (remember, there's basically one for every carbon atom) need to be removed, except for two (this creates the "acid" in fatty acids). With all of the oxygen atoms being released, this leads to a lot of reactive oxygen species ("ROS", aka free radicals), which can wreak havoc on your body. So you're literally using up a lot of electronic energy to store the fat for later.

ONE THING TO keep in mind is that sugar is getting a bad rap these days — more often than not, very justifiably so. You only need small amounts of sugar (less than 5% of total calories is recommended by the World Health Organization), but Western society has become a little bit too keen on the sweet stuff.

How keen are we for the sweet stuff?

Leave it to science to conjure up an interesting experiment. There was actually a relatively recent study (from 2008) comparing the addictiveness of sugar relative to heroin. And guess what? Sugar won. Sugar was found to be more addictive than heroin in those studies. (At least in rats, not people, thankfully; the amount of heroin needed for that would likely have upset the authorities and caused a few social ills.)

Now obviously, we aren't rats. (C'mon now, even those unsavoury lawyers, bankers and politicians aren't rats, however much we might dislike them.) But this does make for a juicy headline. Its truth has been stretched a bit for the sensational headline, but there is a nugget of goodness left there.

Have you ever observed what happens to a veggie tray left out for others? How about a pastry tray? My guess is you've seen what I usually see: the pastries are gone in no time (even immediately after lunch when no one should be hungry), while veggies will sit around all day and likely get tossed. So there is something there with the irresistible pull of sugar.

IT'S no surprise that the food industry is well-aware of our propensity for the sweet stuff. Pretty much everything processed contains sugar. Even things you wouldn't necessarily think of: barbecue sauce, salad dressing, "healthy" cereal, yogurt, etc. However, what's shocking is how some things are touted as "healthy" to make a few more bucks.

As mentioned above, "sugar" is getting a bad rap. And "natural" is all good, right? Honey, maple syrup, agave syrup, rice syrup (brown or otherwise) are all health foods and we can swap these for sugar (or high-fructose corn syrup) without consequence, right?

Not quite.

The natural sugars (honey, maple, rice and agave syrups) are undeniably better for you than refined sugar. But better is an operative word. In the sense that a knife wound is better than a bullet wound.

The rice, agave and maple syrups all contain very small amounts of minerals and other nutrients that are good for you. Personally, I find maple syrup the best of the bunch (certainly taste-wise), but I live in the heart of Maple Syrup Country (yes, capitalised on purpose), so I might be a little biased.

The same goes for honey — yet it also contains small

amounts of protein and enzymes (amazing how good bee vomit tastes, eh? We'll also leave aside the real goodness of royal jelly — honey for the queen bee — which is loaded with nutrients).

Looking a little deeper, honey is still almost pure sugar (about 80% by weight, plus another 17-18% water, so it's at best 3% full of non-sugar nutrients). Because honey is mostly derived from flowers (in other words, fruit precursors, whether it's fruit humans can eat or not), the bulk of the sugar present is fructose, with the remainder glucose and sucrose (which is a combo of fructose and glucose). We'll get into how the body processes fructose a little later.

Maple syrup is about 66% (or two-thirds) sugar, which is almost exclusively sucrose, regardless of grade and another 32% or so of water, so it's at best 1% nutrients. If you've ever had maple syrup, you know that it comes in a few different grades, generally from light to dark, with the darker grades being more flavourful (and also containing more sugar, as more water has been evaporated during processing).

Agave syrup (from the same plant that gives us tequila) is another commonly found natural sweetener. It is about 76% sugar and 23% water, which leaves about 1% of other goodies. What may surprise you is that agave syrup actually has at least as much, and often a bit more, fructose as high-fructose corn syrup (HFCS, about 55% fructose), which is put into just about every processed food. (HFCS is cheap, sweet, and highly profitable, and gets reviled for causing just about every disease known, from diabetes to cancer to dementia.) Remember — fructose gets processed in your body differently than glucose.

In all of these cases, it's clear that you're basically getting sugar water. Small amounts are clearly fine and dandy (and delicious). Just don't think that because they're "all natural" that it's something to eat a cup at a time.

Wanted: FODMAP

No, that's not me being dumb and not knowing how to spell FOOD MAP. But a food map would be a handy thing, right?

FODMAP is short for Fermentable Oligosaccharides Disaccharides Monosaccharides And Polyols... Bit of a mouthful, *n'est-ce pas*? This ties back to the Mr. Potato Head analogy above and the mixing and matching. As discussed above, different carbohydrates/sugars will behave differently in your body.

Some of them are beneficial; some are known to cause bloating and gas. Ever eat too much fruit or too many beans? (I can still sing the lyrics to the song referencing beans as the "musical fruit". Thanks, Dad!) The bacteria in your gut are turning these carbs into gases that cause discomfort for you, and in many cases for those around you, when you release the pressure valves.

What makes matters more confusing is that some people are totally fine with some of these molecules, and others really struggle with them. You literally need to trust your gut on this issue.

For a full list of foods that fall high or low on the FODMAP scale, you can check out: (http://www.monashfodmap.com). They have a great app to help you find what foods are low or high on the FODMAP scale, plus the money you spend goes towards further research into gut health. Win-win!

What's important to know is that a lot of people with suspected gluten sensitivity or intolerance are often eating a fair amount of foods high on the FODMAP scale. By cutting out or greatly decreasing these foods, the gut can heal, and symptoms can improve or disappear. This is not a panacea, but when it comes to your health, even feeling 50% better can make a huge difference in the quality of your life.

So what's the difference between gluten and FODMAP? Gluten is a protein which triggers antibodies to clear it out of your system, while the various sugars get eaten by different bacteria in your gut, creating different products, many of which trigger bloating and discomfort. In many cases, similar effects result (the "get this outta here!!!" effect, aka "the runs"). As someone with Celiac disease, it's really good to know what may be causing the issue and how to prevent things from getting worse. So before you declare all-out war on gluten, see if there might be other foods that are triggering your symptoms. FODMAP might just be the directions you need.

AS YOU CAN SEE, carbs go from simple to complex; at some point, the complexity builds into fibre. Yep, that kind of fibre. This is why fibre is included as a sub-category of carbs in the nutrition fact labels, and is the subject of the next chapter.

4

FIBRE: MORE THAN JUST STUFF TO MAKE YOU POOP

Yond Cassius has a lean and hungry look; He thinks too much: such men are dangerous.

— WILLIAM SHAKESPEARE, FROM JULIUS CAESAR

You may have read *Julius Caesar* back in high school (I did; loved it). Like so many of Shakespeare's plays, there was a solid dose of social commentary and brilliant insight into what makes us tick.

In the play, Caesar is worried about Cassius, who has a "lean and hungry look". He knows well-fed people are not likely to cause him any harm and don't pose a threat to his power. But those lean and hungry ones — watch out!

Things haven't changed since that time. Those who are comfortably off are typically not agents of change — they're much more likely to support the health of the current system. Those who are hungry — they're the destructive ones, the ones who will disrupt the system.

What's true at the societal level is also true at the microscopic biological level. Bacteria present in your gut are no different. If you happen to have a bunch of Cassiuses in there, it's probably a wise idea to make sure they get fed, or prepare to face the consequences.

~

The F Word

Ah... the F word. You were thinking "fibre", right? Right??

Fibre is the new buzzword on the health scene and your doctor might be telling you to eat more fibre.

You may be familiar with Metamucil™, thinking that downing a glass or two of that stuff should help right the ship in the ol' gut, right? Personally, I've never taken the stuff, and it boggles my mind to take an extract of fibre when you can easily get it through something tasty that doesn't come in a bottle — fruits, veggies, nuts and seeds. Surely, somewhere, somehow, you can find a mix that you'll love to eat. Mix it up, too: the more (variety), the merrier (your gut).

So what the heck is fibre, really?

Fibre is the murkiest of those groups on the "nutrition facts" labels. Basically, it's what scientists call the group of food that they weren't able to easily identify back in the early 20th century: "Hey, it's pretty hard to digest and acts like the fibre used to make fabric and clothing, so let's just call it fibre and be done with it." Yeeepppp. Very creative types, those early scientists!

By definition, fibre is what's left over in a food after: (1) extracting any fat in a solvent; and (2) "digesting" the remainder with an enzyme (amylase, which breaks down simple starchy material) and a certain amount of hydrochloric acid (this is the mineral acid present in your stomach; it used to be known as muriatic acid). Fibre is usually classed in among the "carbohy-drate" group, as the bulk of it really is composed of carbohy-drates (or, chemically speaking, linked sugars), plus other goodies like bits of fats, antioxidants, proteins and minerals. In other words, fibre is complex.

The largest bone of contention I have with fibre, however, is that, on nutrition labels, it doesn't count towards the calorie count. To think of fibre as essentially nutrition-free (because it's "calorie-free") will lead to a lot of problems. Remember, calorie content is based on a pretty simple metric that doesn't tell the whole story of how fibre interacts with your body. On the flip side, if you realise that fibre is actually nutrition, then there's enormous gain waiting for you.

Remember how fibre was defined above, and especially how it relates to just the hydrochloric acid and amylase diges-tion? While these conditions are more or less true in your stomach, your stomach isn't where the vast majority of your nutrition gets absorbed. It's your intestines — that's where the magic happens.

If you were to stretch out your intestines (**WARNING!** Do not attempt to remove your intestines to see how long they are, no matter how curious you may be!), you'd easily be able to use them to jump rope. (I also can't recommend strongly enough that you do not attempt to do this either.) All that space in your gut means there's a heck of a lot of bacteria there to either help or hinder your health. You make these bacteria happy by making sure they get lots of good food (fibre, protein, minerals, etc.), and they'll make sure you're in tip-top shape, from head to toe (including the stuff between the ears). Remember, you don't want bacteria behaving like Cassius lurking in your gut.

If fibre really had no calories, as nutrition labels would lead us to believe, then why do your gut bacteria love it so much? Admittedly, some of the fibre will go clean through you, pass GO and collect $200, but a lot will be used by your gut bacteria as food, often to make goodies for you (for example, mood-enhancing serotonin!). We'll cover some of the reasons why you want serotonin in the next chapter on protein.

Another important point: your gut bacteria aren't all the same. They don't all sport the same haircut, wear the same jacket and like the same music. They're different! And do different things! (By the way, they don't actually get haircuts. The jury's still out on the musical preferences.) The key is to have a lot of different good bacteria in your gut, as this will help ensure you have optimal health. Just like nature and society thrive when there's lots of diversity, so does your gut.

The best part is that YOU have a huge say in what bacteria will be hanging out on the inside. You really can starve out bad bacteria and bring in the good ones in a matter of weeks— days if you're prepared to go the biohacker route and ingest fecal implants (in other words, eat poo. Yes, I kid you not, this is a legitimate medical procedure.) This is a case where you feed your gut, and your gut feeds you. To put this another way: You are what you eat.

Gut Bacteria and Why You Want Fibre

As mentioned above, you want the fibre to feed the gut bacteria. Have you ever watched those Snickers commercials where someone gets totally angry/cranky/otherwise very unpleasant? We've even come up with the term "hangry" to describe this situation. I can **definitely** relate to that feeling (or just ask my wife — she insists we bring snacks wherever we go to ward off my hangry side). A lot of gut issues arise when you let them go hungry — in other words, when you don't get enough fibre. They get **hangry**.

Bacteria take out their "hanger" on you by eating up whatever's around them. In most cases, this is the lining of your intestines. If bacteria are eating a hole in your intestines, you're in for a world of pain: leaky guy syndrome, inflammation as your body tries to fight off the bacteria chowing down on the intestinal walls, and more widespread inflammation fighting stuff that isn't meant to be circulating freely in your blood (in other words, the food you just ate).

This is also why highly processed foods are so bad for you; you're literally starving the bacteria in your gut. A lot of the energy of the food has already been released during its processing. This is worse when you eat refined grain flour, as the nutrients have mostly been stripped away before you even get the chance to eat it. It gets even worse: all the remaining energy gets eaten up inside your stomach, so there's nothing left by the time it reaches your intestines and all the bacteria living there. Simple sugars — gone! Lots of flour, especially processed (white) flour — poof! Gone! With nothing left, it looks Cassius is a-coming...

Bacteria are happy little workers, provided they have a paycheque (food) and work to do (break down the food). If you suddenly take away their paycheque, you get some angry bacteria. (Have you ever seen someone happy after getting fired or laid off? Me neither.) Angry bacteria, like angry people, tend to be pretty destructive. Nobody wants that.

As mentioned earlier, you can only get fibre from plants. Fortunately, there are a lot of great plants to choose from. Eating fibre doesn't involve eating grass or hay like a cow would. And you don't have to chow down on tree bark like a beaver. Fruit, veggies, beans/legumes, grains, nuts and seeds all contain fibre. With today's abundance and variety of food, it's pretty close to impossible to not get enough fibre if you pay attention to what you are eating and make some good food choices. Depending on what your current eating habits are like, getting enough fibre might involve getting a little creative or trying out new things, but one thing is for sure: there's something out there that's high in fibre that you like. **You don't have**

to eat kale if you don't want to. If you're on a budget, frozen veggies and fruit typically pack the same nutritional punch as the fresh variety, at a fraction of the cost.

Once you've picked out some new (or old favourite) plant to eat, you can easily find a whole bunch of new and interesting recipes to try out, just by doing a quick search on the ol' inter-webs. While I'm not one to promote herd mentality, most recipes will have reviews, and generally speaking, if the recipe gets at least 4 out of 5 stars, you're usually in good company. Give it a try!

Remember, fibre isn't there just to make you poo. It feeds the bacteria that feed you your vitamins, nutrients and neuro-transmitters like serotonin that literally make you happy. It helps keep you strong, like the topic of the next chapter.

5

PROTEIN: MORE THAN MUSCLES

Great ideas originate in the muscles.

— THOMAS EDISON

*I*n 2008, there was a terrible scandal involving tainted milk in China. A few years' prior, there was a notable increase in rare kidney disease among infants in Gansu province. It became increasingly obvious that the issue was related to something that infants were consuming — in this case, dairy milk-based formula. If you've ever had children, you know that infant diets are pretty limited, so it's relatively easy to pinpoint a cause.

An estimated 300,000 people were affected, including the deaths of six babies and the hospitalization of another 54,000. Virtually all of the victims had issues related to their kidneys.

Because the issue was related to kidneys, the investigators realised that the problem could be related to nitrogen. Kidneys are the main way the body gets rid of excess/waste nitrogen —

by peeing. Urine, while mostly made up of water, also releases urea, which contains two nitrogen atoms, from the breakdown of muscle and other protein-containing molecules.

It was ultimately found that the milk supply had been contaminated with melamine, a molecule containing six nitrogen atoms, thereby giving the illusion that the formula contained more protein than it actually did.

You have probably heard of melamine, or at least one of its products: Formica, the tough-as-nails polymer that is used in most laminate countertops. While it's definitely something that's good for food preparation, it's not something you actually want *in* your food.

Are you thinking, how on Earth can you mistake something that makes hard plastics with protein? Read on.

$$\sim$$

A Rose is a Rose, Except When It's Not

When you read your nutrition labels, you probably think that protein is what it is: protein. Scientists are actually measuring the protein, right?

Nope.

There are indeed methods to measure individual proteins (or rather, their component amino acids). These methods are fairly costly and time-consuming, and require highly-trained personnel. I'm pretty sure none of us want higher food bills just so that we can have a more accurate measure of protein content in our food.

Initially, the main way to measure protein content was a process known as the Kjeldahl method, which relied on a time-consuming, but simple, method and only measured nitrogen (as ammonia). This has now been replaced by a process known as the Dumas method, which is much cheaper and faster: the sample is burned and the nitrogen released is measured, all in a matter of minutes. But in both cases, protein itself is never actually measured; only the nitrogen present in the sample.

This is how the scandal in China came to be. The unscrupulous leaders realised that by doping the milk with melamine, which is very high in nitrogen, they could fake a higher protein content, thereby increasing their profits. Yikes.

Sadly, this falsification for profit still happens, and many milks (dairy or otherwise) are now regularly tested for melamine, as well as protein content.

N is For Protein (and Melamine)

In less frightening news, understanding how protein is measured helps us get the right amount of protein in our diet.

You may or may not have heard claims that you should eat a little bit more plant protein than an equivalent amount of animal protein to get the same amount of bioavailable protein. Unfortunately, those making these statements are a little misguided — it's not entirely that the protein is not bioavailable, it's that, as described above, the tests for protein are measuring nitrogen instead of protein.

It shouldn't come as a shock to hear that plants have a wide range of compounds, many of which scientists haven't "discovered" yet. Some of these compounds will contain nitrogen (N). Remember, the commonly used Dumas method only measures nitrogen, which then gets mathematically converted into protein. So these nitrogen-containing compounds get mislabelled as protein.

As an aside, things like hair, finger and toe nails, and feathers are almost exclusively protein, but we're all aware that they're not something we should be eating. They are not bioavailable: they cannot be broken down or used by the body.

Sadly, most of these things are often contained in processed meats like hot dogs. Ditto for most pet food.

So how is protein actually calculated from the measured nitrogen content? There's a rough factor of 6.25 that is applied to nitrogen to account for the protein content. On *average*, nitrogen makes up about 6.25% of the mass per molecule of an amino acid (with the remainder being carbon, hydrogen and oxygen.) In reality, the nitrogen ratio for amino acids ranges from about 3 to 12, which means you could be getting anywhere from half to twice as much protein as is on the label! Different foods, from animals and plants, will have different amino acids making up their proteins; even the same species grown in different locations and times will have a different composition. As a result, they will have different factors than the 6.25 typically used. Moral of the story: Use the numbers on the nutrition label as a general guide only, and instead try to be in tune with your body, and go by what your body is telling you.

A general rule of thumb is to get about 0.5-1 gram of protein per day for every 0.5 kg (about 1 lb.) of your body mass, or perhaps more appropriately, of the body mass you want to be. Do a rough calculation of what you're getting on a daily basis, then adjust from there. Try getting a bit more if you want to pack on some muscle (or are over 50), or a bit (or a lot) less if you want to shed some weight. Personally, I aim for around 150 g per day. If you eat animal protein (fish, meat), it's really easy to overshoot this. For example, a can of salmon will (according to the label) give you about 45 g of protein, so that alone would give me about a third of my daily requirements. Check back regularly on how you feel and adjust accordingly.

Let's Get Physical

While we are all quite familiar with protein as a building block for muscles, you might not be aware that protein does a lot more than that.

Proteins are actually imbedded in every single cell membrane, typically acting like a transporter of important molecules and nutrients in and out of the cell.

Proteins are also at the "receiving end" of your nerves, and dictate what eventually gets done in the body, although the signals are other molecules. You can think of this like electronic goods; the magic happens when you actually plug things in. Proteins are like the connection at the end that drives what something can do. While electricity travels along wires, it's the connection from the plug to the device that allows things to work.

Protein is also part of the building blocks required to make DNA — in other words, your genes, or what makes you, you (at least physically.)

As I mentioned earlier, protein is actually made up of smaller components, known as amino acids. In total, there are 21 amino acids (at least that are relevant to life as we know it), and humans can only make 10 of them. The others are deemed "essential", or in plain language, you can only get them by eating them! This is the main reason why it's so important to eat a varied diet. Different foods will have different ratios of these amino acids, and we need to make sure we are getting enough of them in our diet.

I won't go through all of the amino acid molecules or names here, but I do want to talk about a certain type of amino acid, called a branched chain amino acid (BCAA). BCAAs have a small portion that makes them less water soluble (hydrophobic, or "water-hating"). This plays an enormous role in how they behave in the body. Their hydrophobic nature means they'll prefer to ball up against any water (the bulk of our bodies), while also "hanging out" with fatty components like the walls of our cells. BCAA also really affect how larger proteins fold together. How proteins fold plays a huge part in how they work. (Or not — diseases like Alzheimer's are known to be to due to protein misfolding.) The branched chain amino acids are leucine, isoleucine and valine. They're the ones required for building muscles, which is why the iron-pumpin' hulks are so intent on supplementing with these specific amino acids.

C'mon, Get Happy!

The goodies from amino acids don't stop there.

As alluded to in the chapter on fibre, part of the reason why we want healthy gut bacteria is because they produce serotonin. Serotonin is known as a mood-enhancing (as in, improving) hormone and neurotransmitter. It's also responsible for regulating our metabolism, whether that's feeling full, or in the event of poisoning from something nasty like *E. coli* bacteria, it fires up the GI Express and gets the bad bacteria out as fast as possible (in other words, you get the runs).

Serotonin is made from the amino acid tryptophan — the same one typically associated with naps on the sofa after a hearty turkey dinner.

ALTHOUGH ANIMAL PROTEIN will have all of the amino acids present in them (known as a complete protein), we need to keep in mind that they are similar to us, in that they get their protein from *their* food. Most of the animals (including many fish) get the bulk of their protein from plants. The more varied their diet, the more likely they will have optimal protein contents as well.

Unfortunately, many animals, particularly those in feed lots or factory farms, are fed a diet consisting primarily of corn and soy. Both of those crops can be grown very economically and can fatten up the animals in a fairly short time leading to larger profits. However, if you've ever eaten a lot of corn yourself, it's pretty obvious that your gut isn't the best at breaking it down. Animals such as cattle are generally much better at breaking it down than people (they do have four stomachs after all!), but the meat produced by a corn and soy diet is of poorer quality nutritionally than that produced by animals that are pasture raised. Pasture raised animals get their protein from a wider variety of sources, which means a more complete profile. They also get a lot more other nutrients, which are then passed on to us.

So no matter how you slice it, it's best to get your protein from a variety of sources, whatever your dietary preferences. We've now covered the big items on the nutrition labels. Now, let's take a dive into the finer details.

PART III

THE DEVIL IS IN THE DETAILS: MICRONUTRIENTS

The devil is in the details.

— PROVERB

Have you ever listened to a webinar or podcast or read a book or blog about a topic you really wanted to learn, and all you got were generalisations, so vague that it might have bordered on useless? With no useful, practical ways to actually achieve a goal?

If you're having any issues with your health, apart from questions related to weight, the odds are changes to your diet could greatly help out your situation.

We all know that it's the small things in life that really bring out the differences. It's these small things that also help us achieve any goal or vision we have for our future. And as the old proverb goes, the devil is in the details.

The small bits are not only harder to see, but they require greater focus to ensure that they serve the greater purpose. As mentioned in the preceding chapters, it's a pretty easy task to figure out how much fat, carbs or protein are present in the food we eat. Figuring out what else is in there not only requires new and better tools, but an entirely new way of looking at your world.

Back in the early parts of the 20th century, scientists developed new ways to analyse specific elements based upon certain properties of these elements. For example, they figured out that sodium emits a yellow light of a particular hue that is unique to sodium when it is burned. This is in part why most streetlights have that yellowish tinge to them— they're based on sodium. (At least until recently with the use of LED light bulbs, which give off different colours and are noticeably brighter.) Methods back then could only analyse one element at a time, so it was extremely time- and resource-intensive to analyse lots and lots of samples. Now, we can analyse over 40 elements simultaneously in a matter of minutes. Not unlike the info on the interwebs, there has been an explosion of info related to elemental composition in foods.

With time, analytical instruments became more sophisticated and more sensitive. What used to be inconceivable is now commonplace. We can now measure every element in the periodic table at levels down to parts per billion and lower (that's 0.0000001% and lower). Because of this, we can now look into how any of these elements behave. It's still really hard, because any single instrument will only give us one point of view— and we need many to really understand what's going on.

In the following chapters, we'll look at the ones we normally find on our nutrition labels (sodium, potassium, calcium, iron), plus some other ones that show up from time to time, but have really significant effects on our health: magnesium, zinc, selenium, copper, iodine and a slew of others. We'll look at how they differ as well as how they sometimes mimic other elements.

6

———

SALT: MORE THAN FLAVOUR

The man worth his salt is the man who meets the needs of the situation in whatever way is necessary.

— Theodore Roosevelt

No matter how good we have it, there's always something we wish was higher, and it has its root in chemistry. What is that thing? Our salary!

Back in Roman times, salt was so valuable that soldiers were paid in salt: their *salarium,* which eventually became the word "salary". Salt was a great form of payment; it was accessible to pay the legions of soldiers, and it was also highly useful for the soldiers and their families.

In fact, there is a lot of evidence that without salt, civilisation would not be what it is today.

For the past several thousand years, salt has been collected from evaporated deposits of salty water, typically from the sea. Salt springs away from the sea arise when water flows through evaporated salt beds from dried up lakes and seas. (The formerly massive Aral Sea, which has all but dried up in my lifetime, will be another one of these salt beds in a few million years.) Salt springs have often led people to dig a little deeper to reveal salt mines.

Salt mines can be found all over the world. In fact, I grew up over one of these salt mines. There is a giant salt deposit under Lake Erie and stretching to the Appalachians. If you are Canadian, you may have purchased Windsor Salt, which comes from the salt mine below Windsor, Ontario (just south of Detroit, Michigan, USA). Sifto salt comes from the same deposit, which happens to be the largest one on the planet. Other popular salts are pink Himalayan salt, which gets its pink colour from trace elements like iron that came from volcanic ash mixed in with the salt, and salt from the Dead Sea, known for its trace mineral content.

Throughout history, towns would often centre around the main industry of salt production, which allowed for trade for other items. In fact, the "wich" suffix in many English towns (for example, Middlewich, Northwich, Sandwich) derived from the fact that salt was produced there: "wich" meant "salt works" in Old English. Salzburg in Austria is another such place, renowned for its giant salt mine.

Salt makes our food taste better; it is, after all, why it's found in every single kitchen, from homes to restaurants, the world over. Salt is also very useful because it can be used to preserve food, as our ancestors knew well. Salt is not just used for encasing a food to dry it out (ham, salt cod). Soy sauce, fish sauce, and fermented foods all require hefty doses of salt. In fact, preservation has been the main use of salt throughout history. Preserving food has allowed us to survive in periods when fresh food is not available, or to travel over long distances, whether by land or sea. Without salt, we wouldn't be where we are today. Clearly, salt has had tremendous value throughout history and is the reason behind the expression "worth their salt". No matter how we look at things, salt is, and will remain, a crucial ingredient in our lives.

WHEN YOU THINK OF SALT, do you think of sodium? Most doctors equate the two. Why is this the case? Most salt is sodium chloride — your typical table salt. Sea salt is also predominantly sodium chloride, plus a lot of trace elements, which we'll cover later in this book. It's also easiest to measure sodium out of all of the components of salt, which is why we generally equate sodium with salt.

In addition to its uses for preserving food and making food taste better, salt is also vital for human life. Sodium and chloride are responsible in part for nerve signalling, which is why we need salt (sodium chloride) to live. Salt, in particular sodium and potassium, is also involved with energy production through the cycling of a molecule known as Adenosine TriPhosphate (ATP) in our cells. Chloride is responsible for balancing electrical charges in the body, helping to ensure proper flow of fluid throughout the body, and is one half of the main component of stomach acid (hydrochloric acid), which helps digest your food. So clearly, getting salt is a necessary thing.

Like anything, however, you can get too much of a good thing. This is what doctors are warning against — getting too much salt, with sodium getting the blame (hence why sodium is on nutrition labels). They know you need salt to live, but we tend to go overboard, especially if you eat a fair amount of processed foods.

So why can sodium be such a menace? Sodium LOVES water. I mean, really, REALLY LOVES water. If you don't believe me, just ask your sweat. Or if you're lucky enough to visit the Dead Sea or Great Salt Lake in Utah, you can see that you can fit A LOT of sodium into a given volume of water.

Sodium will suck up any water that's lying around if you give it a chance. We take advantage of this fact by preserving our foods with it. If you've ever had salt cod, ham or other preserved meat, or even cheese (which is basically salted milk), you'll have noticed its saltiness; salt is the main thing for preserving these foods for consumption later. When you're at risk of starving to death, like many were several generations ago, preserving with salt was a great thing to do to ensure you had something to eat later. Of course, most crackers, chips and other flour-based products are also loaded with salt to keep them shelf-stable for months. Nowadays, however, we have an abundance of food, and we don't really need to do this (no matter how delicious some of these products may be).

Self-Preservation

When we consume too much salt, we are in fact "preserving" ourselves. I put the "preserving" in quotation marks because when things are too salty, they're no longer alive. They just don't rot as fast. So... would you rather be alive, or not rotting as fast?

Aside from absorbing water, another important factor about salt is that extra salt will mess with the consistency of your blood. Your blood is mostly water, but by making it really salty, it becomes thicker, in part because the molecules in your blood start to coagulate, leading to thickening. It's actually a combination of the salt with the organic materials (particularly sugars and proteins) that clump together. If you have ever looked at a river that spills into the sea, you'll see the water go from tea-coloured in the river to clear as things get saltier and the organic, colour-inducing materials clump out. The same principle applies in your veins.

Thicker blood is harder to pump, and blood that is hard to pump, well, can sometimes cause the pump to break from working too hard. You know, that pump called your heart. And I ain't talkin' about the kind of heartbreak you see in movies...

Now, the fantastic part about all of this is that what causes the trouble in the first place is also the solution to the problem (pun intended).

Wait... what?

Sodium (and chloride) is water-soluble, right? As long as you make sure you drink enough water, excessive sodium will likely never be an issue for you. It's just too water-soluble. You'll pee it out. (Over time, however, you will overwork your kidneys if you insist on always eating a lot of salt while drinking gobs of water.)

As we've seen in previous chapters, *correlation is not causation* (everybody repeat after me....). So many health studies have been stymied by the assumption that correlation is causation, when in fact it isn't. Salt (sodium) is used for preserving lots of foods, particularly breads, crackers, prepared meals and deli meats. Because sodium is so much easier to measure than other potentially negative components in food, studies have often linked the higher amounts of sodium in processed foods with negative health effects. But it's not the sodium per se that's causing all of the issues; it's the other stuff that goes along with processed food that's causing the problem. Cut out, or greatly reduce, the amount of processed foods you eat, and you'll likely see some health benefits — and your sodium levels will also drop.

Keep in mind that if you exercise regularly (at least enough to break out in a sweat), you'll be losing lots of sodium, and will need to replenish it.

∼

THE OTHER SALTY element we are going to talk about is potassium.

If you take a peek at the periodic table, you'll see that potassium (K) is directly below sodium (Na). The reason why is that they share a lot of similar atomic properties, and as a result, they behave very similarly. They're both known as important electrolytes (they keep you hydrated and properly functioning) and often do very similar tasks in the body. The trouble is, they're not exactly alike, so if you get too much of one (pretty much always sodium), then your body's function won't work exactly as it should.

Potassium is really important in nerve signalling and a bunch of other important tasks in the body. There's actually a fair amount of research showing that it can help with rheumatoid arthritis. So if you're feeling a little achy in the joints or are having some issues with moving and thinking, getting more potassium (and probably less sodium) could help you out.

The important thing to know is that potassium is needed much more than sodium in the body (and in plants). This is why plants especially tend to have a lot more potassium than sodium. As people, we tend to mess with the sodium/potassium ratios by adding a lot of extra sodium (as salt) to our food. So as long as you eat enough plant foods, you likely won't have too many issues with balancing your sodium and potassium.

Radioactive Bananas?

Bananas are touted as a great source of potassium, which your body needs. However, as we'll cover later, this can lead to a higher dose of naturally-occurring radioactivity in the form of potassium-40! However, unless you go bananas for bananas (like eat 5 or more a day, every day), you've got nothing to worry about.

Sodium is probably the most known dietary element

BONES, MUSCLE CRAMPS AND MENTAL HEALTH: CALCIUM AND MAGNESIUM

To succeed in life you need three things: A wishbone, a backbone and a funny bone.

— REBA MCENTIRE

$\mathcal{B}$ones and calcium are like peanut butter and jam (or maybe peanut butter and chocolate). They go hand in hand.

Bones are loaded with calcium, so it stands to reason that you need lots of calcium to maintain good, strong bones. In fact, of all the ingredients that make up our bones, it's the calcium that is most visible in x-rays; the rest of the stuff is generally pretty dull, which is why it's so easy to see if there are any fractures or breaks in our bones.

The dairy industry has certainly used the calcium-bone connection to their advantage, at least in North America. The North American food guides have always had dairy prominently portrayed as a good source of calcium and necessary for strong bones.

But you know what? They're out to lunch.

Since at least 1999, studies have consistently shown that plant-based sources of calcium are not only higher in calcium, but that your body can actually use this source of calcium. Plant-based calcium tends to stick around, while dairy-based calcium, while containing a good amount of calcium, tends to go through you. In fact, a lot of dairy can actually steal your calcium from you. Osteoporosis is virtually unheard of in cultures that do not consume dairy products, while the rates are considerably higher in cultures that do. Not exactly a promising statistic for encouraging dairy consumption.

I first got interested in this when I became vegetarian (I still ate lots of cheese back then) and thought I had a brilliant plan to test this in the lab — I would show my genius! Alas, a little digging showed that the research had been done a few years prior, and had pretty conclusively shown that it's much better to get your calcium from plant-based sources.

Here's the thing: our bodies are really just a combination of our inputs (food and drink) minus our outputs (no need to be explicit here). Not everything we put in actually gets used (or is "bioavailable"), nor does everything behave the same once inside (this can be both good and bad).

Most of the world can't tolerate dairy, which, up until recently, was purportedly the "best" source of calcium. As I mentioned, osteoporosis is almost non-existent in places of low to no dairy consumption, while in places where dairy is consumed in large quantities, osteoporosis is much more prevalent.

Why is this the case? Milk is relatively high in protein and fat (when whole), both of which are acidic (amino acids and fatty acids, respectively). These acids are great for binding calcium, which means they can bring calcium into your system, but unfortunately, and more importantly, they are also able to take it *out* of your system.

Plants are generally rich in carbohydrates and much lower in protein and fat. Carbs aren't as good at binding calcium, so not only can they release any calcium they've stored more easily, but they're also a lot less able to steal your calcium. Win-win!

If you want to keep osteoporosis at bay, or reduce the risk of making it worse, you will need a good source of calcium, plus a few other things: Vitamin D (we'll cover vitamins later) and the framework that builds the bones, collagen (protein). Oh, and one more thing: magnesium (see below).

Too Much Acid Will Make You a Stoner

No, I'm not talking about that guy who did too many drugs and is now suffering the consequences. But too much acid will make you a stoner of a different kind. We know that acidic compounds can bind calcium. One compound, oxalic acid, is actually two acids in one and binds calcium so tightly that it forms a solid that is really hard to dissolve — in effect, stones. If you've ever had kidney or bladder stones, you know first-hand that they hurt. (Doctors probably don't make things easier by calling them "calculus", in case you didn't already have a negative association with that word from school.)

Do you know what contains a lot of oxalic acid? Potato chips and French fries. (Just in case you needed another reason to avoid them...)

To ensure you don't become a "stoner", the easiest thing you can do is make sure you drink enough liquids, particularly water. With enough water, these stones don't stand a chance of getting big, settling out and causing trouble. Worst case scenario of drinking more water: you get more exercise by going to the loo more often.

O, Mg!

Ever suffer from leg cramps, migraines, or perhaps the threat (real or pending) of osteoporosis? Would you believe there's a single element that could be contributing to all of these symptoms?

If ever you suffer from muscle cramps, especially in your legs, the odds are good that you're missing out on calcium's lighter partner, magnesium (that's the "Mg" in "O, Mg" above).

There's also a lot of research out there showing that people low in magnesium tend to suffer a lot more migraines, both in frequency and intensity. If you've ever suffered from migraines or know someone who has, you know that it's near impossible to get anything done when one hits you.

If you're at risk for osteoporosis, you might want to take a look at magnesium as well. If you're low in magnesium, your body opts for the next best thing: calcium. And as we all know, the main source of that calcium is your bones.

If you're a woman, the odds are much more likely that you have these symptoms than if you're a man. Women are particularly prone to be low in magnesium. Women are also more likely to suffer migraines (about 80% of reported cases). Guess what? In addition to migraines, research shows that magnesium deficiency can also cause depression, which also disproportionately affects women.

Magnesium is also used for energy production in your body. It's a necessary co-factor in the main form of energy generation in all of the cells of your body, from the production of adenosine triphosphate (ATP). So if you're feeling a little sluggish, you might be low in magnesium.

And in case I haven't convinced you yet of the importance of magnesium (particularly if you're female), it's also important for proper nerve, muscle and heart function. In other words, magnesium's got a lot going on!

If you take a gander at the periodic table, you'll notice that magnesium sits directly above calcium. This means it behaves a LOT like calcium. This is important to know because your body is always trying to be in balance, and if you're short on magnesium, your body will look to the next best thing, which is calcium, and start taking a bit from the most abundant source around — your bones. Another thing to keep in mind is that because calcium and magnesium behave similarly, if your diet is loaded with calcium with very little magnesium (likely from a lot of dairy without a lot of veggies, beans and nuts), the (relative) excess of calcium will outcompete any magnesium you do get for the roles that magnesium would normally be playing. Conceptually, you can think of this like any two vehicles that can get you from point A to point B, but if you need to get there fast, you're going to want one with some horsepower. By getting enough magnesium, you'll help your bones stay strong for life, reduce or eliminate muscle cramps and migraines and help stave off depression. O, Mg, indeed!

Between a Rock and a Hard Place

One thing to keep in mind is that the source of the calcium and magnesium you get is very important. For example, you *can* get your calcium and magnesium from rocks (chalk/limestone and Epsom salts, respectively), but I wouldn't recommend trying to eat it to get calcium and magnesium for your body. Here's why: just because a certain amount of those minerals is entering your body, doesn't mean your body can make use of it. Some of the minerals will simply stay in rock form and pass through, meaning that while you did consume it, it's not doing anything for you. Other minerals can have some therapeutic effects when used, yet when consumed, can have a negative effect. Relaxing in a nice hot bath with Epsom salts is great, but if ingested, Epsom salts are great at something else: turning your innards into a GI express train. Not exactly what you want if your aim is to absorb more of your nutritious food.

Ideally, you should be getting all of your calcium and magnesium from food, rather than supplements. If for some reason your doctor recommends that you take supplements of these minerals, make sure they're in an organic (complexed) form. Citrate salts of calcium and magnesium are well-known to be good sources and give you much more bioavailable (biologically useful) forms of these minerals. Now that we've covered two important minerals for keeping you strong, let's look at another, more familiar one.

PUMPING IRON

A true hero isn't measured by the size of his strength, but by the strength of his heart.

— HERCULES

In Greek mythology, Hercules was given twelve seemingly impossible tasks, or labours, as penance for killing his wife and children in a fit of madness. (Soap operas have likely existed since the dawn of civilisation — deep down, we all love crazy stories.) The tasks all involved feats of brute strength in the face of great adversity. Several involved killing mythical beasts like the Hydra (the many-headed serpent), or capturing certain animals. Others were a little less, shall we say, glorious, such as cleaning out the stables of King Augeas in one day, which hadn't been cleaned in 30 years. My guess is that was Herc's favourite. Sure sounds like fun to me.

While the details vary about why certain tasks were given,

how they were accomplished, or who helped whom, one thing is certain: the name of Hercules is synonymous with strength.

WHEN YOU THINK OF IRON, do you think of hulking dudes, overloaded on testosterone, pumping iron while unleashing primal screams as they lift? Like Arnold Schwarzenegger in the 80s?

What if I told you that it's actually **women** who require much higher amounts of iron and that it's women who should be the ones scarfing down those steaks, and not the guys?

It's true. As most women are already aware, menstrual cycles and childbirth burn through iron like there's no tomorrow.

Low iron (anemia) can lead to a bunch of health issues, such as fatigue, weakness, dizziness and lightheadedness. Iron, in the form of haemoglobin, transports oxygen throughout your body. It does this because the form of iron in haemoglobin is able to bind the oxygen you breathe in, then transport it from your lungs and into cells where it is needed. Once inside, the oxygen gets released and is then used for your regular metabolic activities. Without iron, oxygen doesn't bind properly, and only trace amounts make it into your cells. You can think of it like a slow suffocation, as the oxygen you breathe in isn't getting into the cells to carry out their metabolic duties. It's pretty difficult to do just about anything without oxygen. Try not breathing for a minute or more to see what I mean.

Form-idable Strength

Iron comes in lots of different forms. The three main forms are metallic (things like steel and cast iron), ferric iron (Fe^{3+}, think of rust) and ferrous iron (Fe^{2+}, think of blood). The main form your body needs and uses is ferrous iron. This is the iron in haemoglobin (which allows for the transport of oxygen in your blood, and hence, life) and a suite of other important iron-based molecules necessary for life.

The metallic forms aren't really bioavailable, meaning they'll go right through you or just sit there and do nothing. For example, say you were to eat a piece of steel (at least 60% metallic iron). While you would be eating a lot of iron, none of it would be usable.

The ferric forms are somewhat bioavailable, but because they're more oxidised, they don't do the job that iron is usually supposed to do. Ferric ions are in a state of electronic "comfort" and don't want to give up more electrons that are needed to get work done on the cellular level. Ferric iron also requires reduction (aka antioxidants) to become the useful ferrous form, so it can prevent antioxidants from taking care of other, and possibly more pressing, business. In food, you will almost always find the ferrous form. One great source is cacao. That's right. I'm telling you that chocolate (the dark stuff at least) is really good for you and that it's a good idea to eat some regularly. I know, I know — hard advice to follow.

The ferrous forms are the most bioavailable and can generally be put to use by your body right away. If you're supplementing with iron for whatever reason (this will usually be pre- and peri-menopausal women), you need to make sure that the iron is in the ferrous form. The forms most often used are ferrous fumarate and ferrous succinate (in other words, organically-bound iron, not mineral, such as ferrous sulphate). Here's where you really need to pay attention to the labels, as a supplement can be high in iron, but if it's not bioavailable, then you're paying a lot of money for nothing, and that doesn't help your budget or your health. Fortunately, many labels on iron supplements now tell you both the total amount of iron as well as the available amount.

Most people associate iron with beef. They're not mistaken. However, not everyone wants to eat beef, and not everyone should. It uses up a lot of natural resources such as land and water that could be used to do other things like feed more people, clean our air and water, and lead to more natural plant-based medicines.

As mentioned above, a good source of iron is chocolate (yay!), provided it's the dark variety. However, the best source of iron currently known is actually insects like crickets and grasshoppers, as well as mealworms like buffalo worms (beetle larvae). They actually beat out beef by a fair margin when compared on a per gram of protein basis (about 77 micrograms per gram of protein for buffalo worms versus 52 micrograms per gram of protein for beef, or about 1.5x as much). Insect sources are much more economical and environmentally friendly to produce, and if you can wrap your head around eating them, you'll not only get a great source of iron, but protein, too. Full disclosure: I've tried a whole suite of barbecued insects like crickets, worms, and bees; they're delightfully crispy and tasty, like really thin chips/crisps. Insects also are increasingly found in flour form (especially crickets), so you can put them in just about anything without the visuals if that makes you squeamish. I've had a cricket flour protein bar, too. Not as good as the barbecued version, but definitely edible. Again, chocolate is your friend here.

Iron is Rad(ical)

Because iron can be found in several different oxidation states, it can act as a producer of reactive oxygen species (ROS), also known as free radicals. This free radical production happens when the iron "donates" an electron to just about any molecule it comes in contact with in your body to change from the ferrous form to the ferric form (the ferric form being the preferred form to be in). Once a molecule gains that unwanted electron, it becomes a free radical, which can then wreak havoc on your cells by causing a series of chain reactions creating more and more free radicals.

For this reason, although you want to ensure you get enough iron, you also don't want to get too much. So guys, lay off those steaks, alright? Or at least eat smaller portions of them. This is doubly true for those with a condition known as beta thalassemia (where you hyperaccumulate iron), which can be deadly, as all that extra iron leads to extreme levels of ROS that overwhelms the body. Being a little rad is fine; just don't become extremely so.

Iron is clearly necessary for life, but as we've seen, not only do you need the right kind, but you also need the right amount. Next, we'll look at an element that, when combined with iron, makes fool's gold. But this is no fool's errand.

9
———

SULPHUR: SO BAD, IT'S GOOD

Smell is a potent wizard that transports you across thousands of miles and all the years you have lived.

— HELEN KELLER

~

Have you ever walked into a room where garlic and onions were frying and smelled the delicious odour and just started to salivate, imagining how tasty your feast will be? Maybe it's a risotto, or perhaps a delicious Indian dish or a fancy French meal. Mmmmmmm... There's no doubt that your taste buds will be happy.

There's also no doubt that your friends and colleagues will be less than pleased with having a conversation in close quarters with you after you eat such a feast. And definitely not a time for that elevator pitch or important job interview...

Maybe you've been unlucky enough to visit a chicken shed. Ask anyone who's been, and all will tell you that what most call the dreadful rotten egg smell has nothing on a chicken shed.

Or perhaps more interestingly, you are probably familiar with what happens when we relieve ourselves after eating asparagus. Some clever chemists even came up with a unique name for the compound that goes straight to our noses: asparagusic acid. Wherever did they come up with that name?? Just to make us all feel a bit more sophisticated and wealthy, notables such as Benjamin Franklin wrote about the effect asparagus had on his urine in his highly-regarded and erudite essay, *Fart Proudly*. Yes, you read that right. One of the founding fathers of the US, a brilliant scientist and statesman no less, wrote an essay on flatulence. I even have a copy.

Did you know we rely on these smelly compounds to save our lives? All natural gas (the explosive kind, not the kind emanating from our posteriors) is doped with these compounds, so that our sensitive noses can detect if there's a gas leak. Some of you may have allergies to things like mustard, eggs, garlic...Would you believe that a single element is responsible for all of these smells and effects?

Clearly, this chapter is about something smelly. You might even say downright stinky.

All these things have a common cause: sulphur.

Brimstone and Stinging Rain

Sulphur comes in many forms, depending upon its oxidation state. Among the highly oxidised forms are sulphate (SO_4), such as found in Epsom salts (magnesium sulphate) and gypsum (aka gyp-rock, drywall, which is calcium sulphate). You may also be familiar with one of the main causes of acid rain (sulphur trioxide and sulphur dioxide) which are released from combustion of fossil fuels like coal (power plants) and diesel (generators and transport).

Next up, and a little less oxidised, are sulphites (SO_3). Sulphites are reducers (aka antioxidants). You may have seen sulphites as part of the ingredients list on some of the food you buy (like dried fruit) or in that bottle of wine you picked up. As mentioned above, these are antioxidants that help preserve food and prevent wine from becoming vinegar.

However, sulphites can cause a series of health issues. The most common effect is breathing difficulties (asthma), ranging from mild to life-threatening. Less common are rashes and diarrhea.

Sulphur also comes in a reduced form — the infamous rotten egg smell due to hydrogen sulphide that is also a serious health hazard at higher concentrations. The hazard is due in part to it displacing oxygen needed for life (it is a gas after all). The other is its reactivity: hydrogen sulphide reacts quite strongly with many different processes within the body, such as metal (mineral) and protein biochemistry.

Sulphur is interesting in that it can be found in inorganic (discussed above) and organic forms (think biology, not agriculture, when I mention "organic" here). There are two main amino acids that make up the protein in your body: cysteine and methionine. Cysteine is a thiol (which is like an alcohol, but instead of oxygen, has a sulphur atom in its place), while methionine is a thiol ether, meaning there's a carbon group (specifically, a methyl group) on the other end which helps protect the sulphur a bit.

So why does this matter?

The "unprotected" sulphur in cysteine is much more reactive. Generally speaking, this is a good thing. In chemistry, there's a concept of "hardness" and "softness". Basically, "hard" elements like to bind with other "hard" elements, while "soft" likes to go with "soft". It's the "soft" aspect of sulphur that binds to "soft" metals like zinc (important for a lot of healthy things like testosterone production, proper functioning of the lymphatic system to improve and maintaining immunity). It also pulls out toxic metals like mercury and lead, which can either be a good thing or a bad thing (whether those metals are going out of or into your body, respectively).

While having more cysteine can bind more toxic metals (a bad thing), if you limit the amount of metals you're taking in (for example, by cutting back on things like tuna and other top predator fish), then the metals will get diluted and eventually eliminated (particularly in poop) through regular metabolic activity. This is, to quote Martha Stewart, *a good thing*.

Cysteine is one component in glutathione (the other two being glycine and glutamate, or glutamic acid; all components are amino acids). This is one of the most potent antioxidants the body has. Glutathione (and especially cysteine) is also well-known to bind toxic metals like mercury.

Glutathione is responsible for a bunch of beneficial effects in the body, so you'll definitely want to ensure you get enough of its building blocks, particularly cysteine. For metal detoxification, particularly for mercury, lead, arsenic and cadmium, the main way your body detoxifies is through glutathione.

Thankfully, your body is able to make glutathione, so as long as you get the building blocks in your diet, it's not something you might need to supplement with.

You've probably heard lots about the benefits of eating things like broccoli, cabbage, cauliflower and Brussels sprouts. These are all part of the *brassica* family. Brassicas are great sources of sulphur compounds, the same kinds that help detoxify your body of toxic metals.

These compounds actually pack a double-fisted punch. (1) The reduced sulphur is able to act like an antioxidant helping your body in so many ways and (2) they are able to bind and remove toxic metals.

Now remember — your toxic load is a function of not only how many toxins you take in during a given time period, but also how quickly you can get rid of them. By eating things like the brassicas, you can speed up how quickly your body gets rid of these toxic compounds. Not only are they rich in these great sulphur-containing compounds, but they're also rich in fibre. And we all know what eating a lot of fibre does... It makes those gut microbes happy and gets rid of junk in the body! Woohoo!

Unfortunately, the brassicas often get a bad rap. They're pretty distinct, flavour-wise. They require a fair amount of chewing if eating them raw. If, like me, you only had them boiled to death when you were younger, then yeah, I agree, they're not something that makes you ask for more (or any!).

However, if things like broccoli, cauliflower, and Brussels sprouts turn you off, try roasting them. My young kids actually ask for them, and can't get enough. (Seriously. We were shocked, too.) Toss the broccoli in some soy/tamari sauce and sesame oil. Cauliflower just needs olive or avocado oil and salt, and the Brussels sprouts just need oil, salt and maybe some diced onion. For any of these, roast them on a cookie sheet around 200°C (375°F) for 15-20 minutes (or a bit more if you like it kinda crispy or a bit more of the delicious browning). Just because it's healthy, doesn't mean it can't taste great. Great taste *AND* healthy? Sounds like a win-win to me.

Sulphur isn't the only element to have a number of useful forms. We'll cover a few more in the next chapter.

10

MULTI-TALENTED ELEMENTS: SELENIUM, ZINC, AND COPPER

The food you eat can either be the safest and most powerful medicine, or the slowest form of poison.

— ANN WIGMORE

Hopefully the preceding chapter convinced you of the benefits of eating smelly food (beyond being able to fend off vampires). Sulphur compounds are indeed really good for you. But so is another similar element, and it's found just below sulphur in the periodic table. And it has something to do with Star Trek. (Just go with me on this one.)

If you've ever seen Star Trek (the original version with William Shatner and Leonard Nimoy), you'll know that you don't want to mess with Dr. Spock. Why not, you ask? Is it his superior intellect and emotionally-remote logic?

No. It's the fearsome Vulcan Death Grip.

Spock's Death Grip got the crew of the USS Enterprise out

of a few sticky situations. I would argue that there's an element that does just this: selenium.

Selenium's grip on certain metals is basically a Vulcan death grip. Because of this, selenium is great at detoxifying heavy metals, particularly mercury. Remember the hard-soft concept in the previous chapter? Well, selenium is even "softer" than sulphur. As a result, it has a Vulcan death grip on mercury. Want to drop your mercury levels as soon as possible? Make sure you eat something with selenium in it.

Selenium is also involved in several processes related to cancer suppression and good cardiovascular function, primarily from its ability to be in several different oxidation states, several of which are antioxidants. Like sulphur, selenium can be in several different oxidation states. Because of this, the form you actually consume is really important. At the low end (most reduced), selenium behaves just like the sulphur in things like cysteine and glutathione. Again, scientists got really creative and named these compounds selenocysteine and selenoglutathione. (Their creativity knows no bounds!) These compounds do more or less what their sulphur cousins do, but generally better (or at least, faster).

Selenium also comes in more oxidized versions (beyond metallic selenium): selenite and selenate. Because selenite can still be oxidized, it's still an antioxidant, plus it's easier for that to be turned into the reduced selenium compounds mentioned above (win-win!). If you do happen to supplement with selenium, or see it on your label, try to make sure it's either the selenite (usually as sodium selenite) or reduced form of selenium (typically the selenocysteine and selenoglutathione compounds mentioned above).

So that's all fine and dandy, but where can we get selenium besides from a chemical lab?

Most nutritionists will tell you to go to Brazil and eat their eponymous nut. Brazil nuts are indeed high in selenium, as they suck up a bunch of the selenium present in the soil. (Selenium, like gold and oil, isn't distributed evenly throughout the planet. Brazil just happens to be one of those places with lots of selenium.) However, the devil is in the details here.

You definitely need selenium in your diet for optimal health. However, the optimal range is pretty narrow. When you go beyond this, you can develop what is known as selenosis (yes, one of those dreaded "osis" things). Trust me — you don't want selenosis. Besides the fun involved with nausea, diarrhea and fatigue, you also get to enjoy hair and nail loss and general internal hemorrhaging. I'm not sure about you, but that's convincing enough for me to avoid getting too much selenium.

Back to Brazil and those nuts.

Depending on where they're grown (even within Brazil), Brazil nuts can range from relatively low amounts of selenium, to super-high amounts that would do serious damage to you if you ate one or two of them regularly (as in, at least once a day). In fact, concentrations varied by as much as 500x in one recent study from Brazil. It's these high levels that make selenium go from friend to foe.

Now I know that you're not going to research exactly where your Brazil nuts were grown and compare that with levels of selenium found in those soils, nor are you going to run samples of every nut you eat to make sure you fall within a safe zone of selenium consumption. (This would be a case of you are what you eat: a nut.) However, if you eat one nut a day, you should be safe. My recommendation would be to store them in the fridge or freezer — and buy as fresh as possible — because Brazil nuts go rancid pretty quickly, which defeats the entire purpose of eating them for their antioxidant properties.

~

It's Not What You Zinc

We hear loads of press about sodium, calcium, and iron. They are certainly required (within limits) for life. As covered in the preceding chapters, each of these has specific roles to play in the body. Yet none of these is involved in every single process in the body.

While we might be tempted to think metals (minerals) are only good for very specific tasks and nothing else, this isn't always the case. There actually is a metal that is involved in all of our bodily processes. Chances are, you haven't heard of it.

So, to paraphrase JRR Tolkien's *The Lord of the Rings*, what is this element that unites them all?

Zinc.

You might be more familiar with zinc than you think. It's one of the two main components in brass (the other being copper). It's also used "head and shoulders" above other active ingredients in anti-dandruff shampoo and as the anti-bacterial ingredient in certain dishwashing sponges. (Those sponges still get loaded with bacteria anyway, which is why you should replace them on a regular basis.) However, these uses are all designed to prevent (microbial) life from taking over. What actually makes it indispensable to life?

Zinc is indispensable to pretty much every facet of life for us, from reproduction and growth to immunity to learning. Not only is it necessary in over 300 enzymes, but it's also involved with over 1000 transcription factors (this relays "information" in the body by turning genes on or off as necessary). Zinc is used for muscle growth and maintenance by way of programmed cell death, or apoptosis, which helps keep things like cancer in check. It's involved in a lot of immune system functions, which is why it's so highly touted for getting over colds — you'll still get them, they'll still suck, but they won't last as long. It also helps the brain remain "plastic", which means keeping it able to learn new things and "young". In other words, zinc is kind of a big deal.

The best sources of zinc are usually from animals, especially oysters (they lead the pack by a fair margin). If you're not inclined to eat animals, you can still get enough zinc from your diet. The catch is that zinc in plant-based sources might not be so bioavailable. Plants, especially nuts and seeds, use a compound called phytic acid to concentrate phosphorus (that's one of the main ingredients in fertilisers). Phytic acid, or phytate, is amazing at grabbing elements like calcium, magnesium, iron and zinc and holding on pretty tightly, meaning it'll go right through your body, without releasing the goodies.

However, if you get too much zinc, it messes with copper, which we'll look at next.

$\sim$

Coppers and Robbers

It's funny how we don't really value what is most useful to us. Of the three coinage metals (copper, silver, and gold), the least valuable of the coinage metals is also the most important in our lives. If you live with indoor plumbing and electricity, you rely on copper. Most pipes are made with copper, as are electrical wires (the conducting part, at least). Copper, in the form of brass (an alloy with zinc), is also used heavily in marine hardware, as it won't corrode easily. If you get anything by sea (which means you don't live like a caveman or live strictly off the land on which you live), you rely on copper. You might even have some copper pots and pans in your kitchen.

Copper's usefulness extends beyond the industrial. If you're a fan of music, you're a fan of copper — it's integral to brass, which makes most wind instruments. If you're an art afficionado, you might also enjoy bronze sculptures. Bronze is a copper alloy.

Clearly, copper is very versatile. What might surprise you, however, is how versatile it is in our bodies.

Mining the Motherlode

Believe it or not, we start our lives with the highest amount of copper we'll likely ever have. Fetuses in the last trimester go on a copper spree and suck up all they can from their mothers, storing up the copper in their livers. Why are fetuses so hungry for copper?

Copper is needed for a bunch of growth-related processes, from bones to muscles and connective tissue to the cardiovascular system to the brain. In other words, pretty much everything. So you can see why babies are so hungry for copper.

Copper can also act as an antioxidant. How does it do this? Copper (Cu) prefers to be in a divalent, or cupric form (as Cu^{2+}; think of the green metal roofs as the red copper metal corrodes and oxidises). The other favourable oxidation state is cuprous, or Cu^{1+}. The main difference here is that the cupric form is much more important in the body. The cupric form is typically the one that's found in many important enzymes. What's more, cupric copper can absorb an electron from free radicals. When it does this, it transforms into the cuprous form and neutralises the free radical. Woohoo!

So where can you get copper?

You can get small amounts from the water you drink, assuming you have copper pipes in your home. However, most of it will come from your food. The wider the variety, the better.

Good sources are seafood (especially shellfish like lobster), beans and nuts, whole grains like wheat and rye, organ meats (especially liver) and best of all, chocolate. I mean, can there ever be too many reasons to eat chocolate? So go ahead, indulge a little. For your health.

The elements covered in this chapter help out your immune system. We'll cover another one in the next chapter that's a bit more targeted in its effects.

11

———

IMMUNITY AND YOUR THYROID:
IODINE

Healing is a matter of time, but it is also sometimes a matter of opportunity.

— HIPPOCRATES

Fatigue. Joint pain. Difficulty shedding extra weight. Brain fog. If you have issues with your thyroid, you may be experiencing any or all of these conditions. And if you're a woman, you're three times more likely than a man to develop thyroid-related symptoms.

Autoimmune diseases related to the thyroid appear to be increasing. Hashimoto's disease, Graves' disease, and hypothyroidism are some of the diagnoses increasingly being heard linked to symptoms of fatigue, pain and difficulty losing weight. Surprisingly, even though there's a huge amount of things that your thyroid does for you, a lot of your thyroid's activity relies on just one element: iodine.

So what exactly does iodine do?

Iodine helps regulate your immune system. There are two significant compounds in iodine: triiodithyronine and thyroxine. To make things easy, science has decided to call them T3 (triiodithyronine) and T4 (thyroxine). They look like this:

$$\text{L-Thyroxine (T}_4\text{)}$$

$$\text{3,5,3'-Triiodo-L-thyronine (T}_3\text{)}$$

As you can see, T3 has three iodine (I) atoms in the molecule, while T4 has four. Brilliant naming scheme, right?

What's really important is that the thyroid controls a lot of how your body processes metabolic activity. Depending on levels of T3 and T4 and the related hormones TRH and TSH, you may either be burning a lot of calories with ease or having a really hard time burning those calories off. The thyroid also controls your heartbeat and how your muscles contract (which includes moving food through your gut). So to make sure that your thyroid works as it should, eat some iodine.

The main sources of iodine in your diet are sea salt (in trace amounts) and seaweed such as dulse or nori (some table salts are also iodised, and will say so on the package). These are excellent sources of iodine. As you may have noticed, both sources are from the sea.

Thankfully, you don't *have* to live by the sea to get this important nutrient, although it sure would be nice to do so.

Clearly, the easiest route for iodine intake would be to salt your food with sea salt. Just remember — you don't need a huge amount, and as we covered earlier, the goal is to add the necessary salts (including iodine) to your body, not to preserve your body like ham. Personally, I find most varieties of seaweed very tasty, and *might* have polished off a roll or two (or thirty) of sushi in one go on more than one occasion.

Iodine and Radioactivity

If you had to choose to get cancer, you would probably want to get thyroid cancer. What is interesting, however, is that women are three times more prone than men to getting this type of cancer. Obviously I wouldn't wish this on anyone, but the odds for recovery are quite favourable. Recovery rates due to advances in medicine now put cure rates at at least 90%.

So how come recovery rates are so high with this type of cancer? One word: radioactivity. Nuclear medicine (aka radio-pharmaceuticals) is what saved the day. Radioactive isotopes behave pretty much the same as stable isotopes. Iodine goes straight to the thyroid, and radioactive iodine can only impact a distance of up to 2 mm (less than 1/12th of an inch). So we can use radioactive iodine (typically I-131) to help destroy any cancerous tissues in the thyroid, and the rest of the body can stay healthy. On the flip side, regular iodine is also how we get rid of radioactive iodine. If ever there's a nuclear attack or accident at a nuclear power plant, potassium iodide (KI) pills are given out to help counteract any radioactive iodine that is released. (Iodine is a fission, or breakdown, product of uranium in reactors.) If you ever see "iodized salt" on a package of salt, it just means that some KI has been added to it.

Now that we've covered some of the more common elements in your body, let's delve a little deeper into some of the lesser known ones.

12

CORNUCOPIA OF TRACE ELEMENTS

It's the little things that count.

— PROVERB

∾

Useful, and Toxic, Chromium

If ever there was an element associated with an individual who wasn't involved in its discovery, that element would be chromium and that individual would be Erin Brockovich. Many of you may have seen the movie from 2000 starring Julia Roberts portraying the environmental activist.

So what was all the fuss about?

Erin Brockovich noticed that there was a higher incidence of certain cancers in a region in California. She also noticed that water in the region contained an element known to be toxic: chromium. The Erin Brockovich hexavalent chromium case is one of the worst offenders on the misuse of statistics, affected by ignorance of sampling bias in a small area and without regard to rates found elsewhere. However, the upside is that other areas with much higher levels of chromium were discovered, leading to improved health for many people.

It's important to note that one form of chromium, known as hexavalent chromium, is responsible for most of the toxicity. "Hexavalent" refers to the fact that this form of chromium (Cr) is short six electrons from its metallic form, giving it an oxidation state of +6. (The metallic form of chromium is the kind that gives cars that shiny metallic look, which we typically call chrome). Chemistry geeks like me know it as Cr^{6+}.

The reason Cr^{6+} is so toxic is because it's really easy for the chromium to rip electrons out from other elements or compounds (like those in your body) in order to return to a different oxidation state: Cr^{3+}, or trivalent chromium. Remember, it's short six electrons, and prefers to be in the trivalent form, so Cr^{6+} will take those electrons where it can find them.

Trivalent is the other common form of chromium. Trivalent chromium is the type of chromium that is actually required in certain biological processes. Research has shown that, in trace amounts (10s of parts per billion, or about 0.000001%), we need chromium to help with proper insulin function. Insulin is probably one of the best known hormones, and it helps us metabolise (or store) carbohydrates, fats and protein. So if you suffer from diabetes or know someone who does, you might want to get your chromium levels checked.

While you can supplement with chromium, keep in mind the most bioavailable sources are based on organic compound complexes (typically as picolinate or Glucose Tolerance Factor (GTF)). Other forms (say, chromium chloride) are essentially useless. Your body can't make much good use of it, so it's important to read the label. Clearly, the best way to get chromium is in food. Broccoli and red grapes appear at the top of the list, but most foods have trace amounts, that when combined, will give you enough. Just avoid simple sugars; these tend to send chromium straight through your gut and out the other end.

Larry, Curly and Mo(lybdenum)

Decades ago, when scientists were still trying to figure out everything that went on in nuclear reactors, they kept discovering new fragments (called "daughters") that were being produced from fission (splitting apart) of uranium. One of these daughters, or fission products, was molybdenum. The form of molybdenum produced by fission, Mo-99, eventually decays into the lightest man-made radioactive element, technetium (Tc). Technetium is interesting because it's the only element (beyond the really heavy ones like plutonium) that doesn't exist in nature.

Technetium is also used extensively in medicine and has saved hundreds of millions of lives (and counting). Have you ever had to get a PET or CT scan? If so, you may have had to ingest some technetium. Both PET and CT rely on radioactive isotopes like technetium, so molybdenum plays a critical role in a lot of diagnoses. There's definitely some pretty interesting science going on with a PET or CT scan that allows to see what you look like on the inside, from bones to organs and everything in between. But molybdenum is required for more than just nuclear medicine. Its stable isotopes are also required for life.

Have you ever looked at a multi-vitamin bottle and seen "molybdenum"? Rest assured that this won't be the radioactive version. Ever wonder what the heck it is?

Molybdenum (Mo) is just below chromium on the periodic table. Like chromium, molybdenum has a number of different forms it can take, and most involve some really nice colours. Like chromium, you really only need very small amounts of molybdenum — micrograms, in fact. (A microgram is about the weight of an eyelash.)

Molybdenum is important in a number of biological processes. It's critical for the metabolism of sulphur-containing amino acids like methionine and cysteine. Without the metabolism of these amino acids, numerous neurological issues result, such as brain wasting (atrophy) and seizures. Molybdenum helps to rid your body of toxins and drugs. It also ensures that your blood has a certain amount of antioxidant capability.

Molybdenum deficiencies are rare and usually linked to areas with poor amounts in the soil. The best food sources are beans, lentils and peas, followed by nuts and grains. Animal products and fruits and veggies are generally low in molybdenum.

Nope, Not That One...

Another important micronutrient is manganese (not to be confused with magnesium). Manganese sits right next to chromium in the period table of elements. Like chromium, manganese also has a variety of oxidation states, ranging from metallic (oxidation state of zero, or "zero-valent") to higher oxidation states (usually found as oxidation states of 2, 4 and 7, with each manganese oxidation state having a distinct colour). In fact, manganese in the highest oxidation state, in compounds like potassium permanganate, can be used as a cleaning agent for wounds, as it's a really strong oxidant (not unlike iodine). (Side note: if ever you find yourself alone in the woods and need to make a fire, add a little permanganate to a pile of something organic, like some dried leaves or bits of fat, and voilà! A little fire will start without too much effort.)

What's great about manganese is that because it can have so many different oxidation states, it's a wonderful antioxidant. It's even a crucial component in the superhero-sounding enzyme manganese superoxide dismutase. The name says it all, right? This manganese enzyme transforms ("dismutes", or mutates away from) superoxide, which is a very potent reactive oxygen species, or more simply, a very strong oxidant (which is why we're encouraged to consume lots of antioxidants; see Chapter 14 for more on antioxidants). This enzyme is especially useful in the energy factories of our bodies (mitochondria), as they produce lots of superoxide from oxygen when they make energy in the form of ATP, the main molecule responsible for energy transfer in the body.

Depending on the oxidation state, manganese is used in a variety of enzymes that help with metabolism of carbohydrates, protein and cholesterol. It also helps with bone formation, in particular collagen (the organic framework of bones and cartilage).

If you eat mostly plants, you'll get all the manganese you need. Good sources are nuts, leafy greens and whole grains. Tea is a surprisingly good source, as well.

We've covered the important parts of the periodic table. Next, we'll look at the other items on nutrition labels: vitamins and antioxidants.

PART IV

THE ALPHABET AND THE RAINBOW: VITAMINS AND ANTIOXIDANTS

13

VITAMINS

Curiosity is the vitamin of learning.

— SIR KEN ROBINSON

~

What You Eat Matters

We've all been told since we were children to take our vitamins; that they're good for us, etc.

The most popular vitamin is probably Vitamin C. So... if you had to guess where you should get Vitamin C from, what would you say?

Oranges? You wouldn't be alone.

The orange industry has certainly convinced many of us that the best source of Vitamin C is oranges. There is definitely Vitamin C in oranges. But guess what? Vitamin C is in a lot of other foods, too, and usually in higher quantities than in oranges.

What's really important, however, and something that has

been missed altogether in lots of medical advice, is that vitamins are something found *in* food. In other words, they actually work best when coupled with the right food. Vitamins need to be in the right environment for them to work properly.

What do I mean by this?

Vitamins can be divided into two main groups: water-soluble and fat-soluble. For a water-soluble vitamin to work, it needs to be in water. Our blood is mostly water (as is most of our body), so this is pretty easily done. It also means that we can easily pee them out if we happen to take too much of one of them. By the same token, we have to ensure we get a consistent supply of these vitamins, because, well, we pee them out.

On the other hand, fat-soluble vitamins require —*gasp*— fat. Without adequate fat, consumed at the same time as the fat-soluble vitamins, these vitamins won't do you as much good. So you could be taking your vitamins (in pill form) with religious fervour every single day, but if you aren't eating fat at the same time, you're really not getting the best bang for your buck. Fortunately, most fat things are delicious — nuts, seeds, avocados, oils, and yes, animal fat, too. If you happen to take your vitamins with your breakfast, make sure you're also eating some fat.

Because fat-soluble vitamins dissolve in fat, they're able to stick around a little longer, as our cells are completely surrounded in fat. Since they can stick around longer, we're able to store them up a bit, so it can become a problem if we load up on vitamin supplements of the fat-soluble variety. If you get your fat-soluble vitamins from your food, the odds are really good that you won't have any such issue.

Know Your ABCs

Since you are reading this book, I'm pretty confident you know the alphabet. So let's look at our (vitamin) ABCs, okay?

Unfortunately, there's no rhyme or reason to the letters scientists have associated with all of the vitamins. The following table lists all of the vitamins and divides them into the fat-soluble and water-soluble groups.

Water-soluble Vitamins	
B1	Thiamin
B2	Riboflavin
B3	Niacin
B4	Choline
B5	Pantothenic Acid/Pantothenate
B6	Pyridoxine/Pyridoxamine
B7	Biotin
B9	Folic Acid/Folate
B12	Cobalamin
C	Ascorbic Acid/Ascorbate
Fat-soluble Vitamins	
A	Retinol/Retinal/Retinoic Acid
D	Cholecalciferol
E	Tocopherol
K	2-methylnaphthoquinones

From the table, you might think that scientists don't know how to count or spell. (What happened to 8, 10 and 11, or F through J?) In any case, the letter and numbering system is just a simplification. Who needs to spend the extra mental calories remembering those names anyway? You have more important things to focus your mind on.

If you want to simplify things a step further, just know that B and C vitamins are water-soluble, and everything else is fat-soluble. Three simple facts. Not so bad, right?

Vitamins are found in all sorts of food, in varying amounts, so by eating a lot of different foods (with and without high fat content), you should be able to get all the vitamins you need. One caveat: if you're vegan, it can be really hard to get enough Vitamin B12, which is typically only found in animal sources (only trace amounts are found in plants). That said, in all cases, it's bacteria that produce it. So finding a source that works for you (which can be in supplement form) should solve any problems with getting enough.

Eating a wide variety of foods is clearly needed to get all of your vitamins; it's also necessary for the class of compounds in the next chapter.

14

ANTIOXIDANTS

Try to be a rainbow in someone's cloud.

— Maya Angelou

You've no doubt heard a whole bunch about antioxidants and how you should be consuming more of them to improve your health. But not all antioxidants are good for you. That's right — some antioxidants are downright nasty!

How can this be?

Getting a little nerdy with some chemistry, antioxidants are compounds that oxidise more easily than some nutrients you want for good health (like omega-3 fatty acids). Since they react more readily with oxidisers, antioxidants become oxidised, sparing some more important compounds (like the fat making up our cell membranes, our DNA... you get the idea). So basically they sacrifice themselves so that what we want for our health can be preserved. And yes, I chose the word "preserved" on purpose. Preservatives *are* antioxidants. Yet, we generally want our food to be free of preservatives.

So what's the difference?

There are a couple of differences, actually.

There are organic (as opposed to inorganic, or "mineral") antioxidants, such as those found in fruits and vegetables. Organic antioxidants tend to have similar structural features to one another. Given these structures, organic antioxidants are more able to penetrate into cells and have a wider effect on health by taking out the free radicals from reactive oxygen species (ROS), reactive nitrogen species (RNS) and reactive sulphur species (RSS). Generally speaking, you don't want a lot of ROS, RNS or RSS, as the radical can lead to a destructive chain reaction until it finally reacts with something that can stabilise it (like those antioxidants!). The reason why it's good to eat a wide range of colourful produce is that the pigments in these foods have the chemical structure that works wonders at stopping those ROS in their tracks.

Remember how vitamins come in water-soluble and fat-soluble forms? Guess what? Antioxidants follow the same pattern.

Let's look at two colourful root vegetables: carrots and beets. Carrots are usually a bright orange colour due to the pigment beta-carotene (which is where the name originated from — carrots!). If you've ever cooked carrots in water (steamed or made into soup), you'll notice that the carrots tend to keep their orange colour and not really colour the water orange (assuming you keep them whole). Now look what happens with beets — you get a rich reddish-purple colour in the water right away, plus it stains your fingers when chopping them.

So what's going on?

Water-Soluble

Water-soluble antioxidants are generally in what's known as the polyphenol form, or simply polyphenols. An example is something such as the anthocyanins. Foods containing anthocyanin include blueberries, red/purple grapes, raspberries, red cabbage, etc. In other words, reds, blues and purples. The antioxidant part of anthocyanins and other polyphenols is due to the phenol groups of these molecules. They act as antioxidants by sucking up reactive oxygen species (ROS), and other related compounds known as free radicals. They're also good at absorbing UV radiation, which would otherwise damage important molecules, like your DNA.

There is another group of water-soluble antioxidants known as the betalains. (Or perhaps more appropriately, "bee-talains", as they were first discovered in beets.) These are more frequently reds, oranges and yellows. Beets, chards and other leafy greens with red, orange or yellow tinges are rich in beta-lains (and don't contain any anthocyanins). While these often contain phenol groups, their structure and behaviour is different from the anthocyanins — their colour is due to what is known as conjugation, which is unsaturated fat-like components. In particular, betalains are much more water-soluble. If you've eaten a lot of beets, you may have noticed that your pee turns a little reddish. And if you get beet juice on something, it is also a lot easier to wash off the colour than it would be for something like blueberry juice.

Fat-Soluble

Beta-carotene is a fat-soluble antioxidant so it won't dissolve much in water. (It's often used in imitation butters to give the yellow colour normally found in butter.)

You may have also heard of lycopene. It's almost identical to beta-carotene, but instead of the orange associated with beta-carotene, lycopene is bright red. Tomatoes owe their red colour to lycopene.

Lutein is another fat-soluble antioxidant that is very structurally similar to beta-carotene.

And curcumin, the most prominent pigment in turmeric, is also fat-soluble. Curcumin has this beautifully symmetrical structure:

The molecule is actually perfectly symmetrical: the "O" and "OH" in the middle "share" the hydrogen (H). The few oxygen atoms present mean that the molecule is barely soluble in water. This is why both nutritional scientists and Ayurveda practitioners recommend you eat fat when you have turmeric; it needs the fat to help it move into cells. Curcumin is touted as having a lot of great health benefits, such as reducing inflammation (which is great for arthritis!), headaches, gastrointestinal issues and possibly helping with mental decline as we age.

Your body is basically water and fat. Combined, your body is at least 75% of these two components. Because of this, it's really important to eat both types of antioxidants so that they can access all parts of your body. This is why it's recommended to eat a wide variety of colours, from the oranges and reds all the way through to the purples. As the Skittles commercial used to go: eat the rainbow. (Just not in candy form!)

~

THERE ARE ALSO INORGANIC ANTIOXIDANTS, such as sulphites and nitrites. These would typically be called preservatives. If you haven't noticed these compounds when you read a label with these compounds in them, you probably will now!

Sulphites are used particularly with dried fruit, wine, and other preserved foods, while nitrites are used mainly with meat, especially beef. Nitrites are loaded in most hot dogs and cuts of beef. In fact, the reason why the beef looks more appealing (and red) at the grocery store is because of the presence of nitrites. Without them, the surface of the meat would oxidise and turn brownish. As a consumer, you're not likely to pick up a piece of uncooked brown meat, are you?

Unfortunately, these compounds are increasingly being shown as having an array of negative effects on the body, including cancer. In addition, although these preservatives don't make their way into cells all that well (they're very water-soluble), they are much more potent than the organic antioxidants listed above.

PART V

THINGS TO AVOID

15

____

TOXIC METALS: ARSENIC, LEAD, AND MERCURY

You're a foul one, Mr. Grinch! You really are a heel! You're a three decker sauerkraut and toadstool sandwich...with arsenic sauce!!!

— Dr. Seuss

Why Rice Might Make You a Grinch

A Christmastime tradition in my family is to watch Dr. Seuss' *How the Grinch Stole Christmas*. If you've ever watched *How the Grinch Stole Christmas* — the original cartoon one, that is — you've probably heard the great songs describing the mean, old Grinch and likening him to a not-so-appetising sauerkraut and mushroom sandwich with "arsenic sauce".

Obviously, no one wants to be a mean, old Grinch, but it might not be that easy to avoid being filled with arsenic sauce.

Wait, what!?

It all comes down to whether or not you eat rice, and where that rice came from.

Rice grows in paddies that are submerged in water. When things are submerged in water, the oxygen concentration drops dramatically. The air you breathe is about 20% oxygen, yet highly oxygenated water is only about 8-10 parts per million (ppm) oxygen, which is 0.001% (at best). In other words, the amount of oxygen in water is at least 20,000 times lower than the amount in air. Warmer water has even less oxygen, and most things living in water, including bacteria, use up the oxygen pretty quickly, so the oxygen concentration will often be less than 1 ppm (0.0001%). Rice paddies fall into that 1 ppm or less category (what the science folk call "anoxic" or "suboxic").

But back to the arsenic sauce…

Arsenic is one of the elements that can take many forms (oxidation states). These different forms have different health effects and different behaviours in the environment. Completely oxidised arsenic (the +5, or pentavalent, oxidation state) is not very soluble and will stay stuck to certain minerals, especially iron oxides (basically rust). This form will be present when there's enough oxygen around (such as in moving water like rivers). This is a good thing, as there's loads of iron available to suck up the nasty arsenic.

However, this form of arsenic can also mimic the phosphate group. Phosphate is involved in things like metabolism and energy exchange (you may have heard of adenosine triphosphate, or ATP, as the major mover-and-shaker for energy in the body). Arsenic (As), as arsenate (AsO_4), has the same general formula and "shape" as phosphate (PO_4), and is actually found just below phosphorus in the periodic table, which allows it to mimic that important phosphate group, without giving the same benefits. In other words, arsenic (+5) can have some negative health effects as it messes with these metabolic processes.

The other main form of arsenic is the slightly reduced form (+3, or trivalent, oxidation state). This form occurs in areas with really low oxygen levels such as those found in rice paddies. It is also much more water soluble than the +5 form. As paddies get flooded, arsenic that may have been in the +5 form gets reduced to the +3 form, released from the rocks and minerals it was bound to, and can then get taken up by rice during its growing period. In places like Bangladesh where there is a lot of arsenic in the ground, the use of groundwater for rice cultivation is making matters really bad, as the flooding is leaching out the arsenic from the ground and rocks below and into the rice.

Long story short, if you eat a lot of rice, particularly rice grown in an arsenic-rich region, you stand a good chance of getting arsenic poisoning. And no one wants to be a Grinch.

Of Energy and Impostors: Cadmium

Besides their use in batteries (nickel-cadmium), you probably haven't heard much about cadmium. However, it is a toxic element. Why? Let's have a look at the periodic table again.

Remember the chapter on zinc, specifically how zinc is responsible for a whole series of positive health effects, like growth and immunity? Cadmium sits directly below zinc on the periodic table. This means that cadmium is also able to mimic zinc in many cases. This is yet another case of where mimicry is bad.

Instead of being in the Goldilocks zone for proper function, cadmium is bit more like Papa Bear — a bit too big. As a result, biochemical processes that rely upon zinc don't work when cadmium substitutes for zinc, and we don't get the growth and immunity we need.

What makes matters worse is that cadmium actually binds *more strongly* than zinc to sulphur-containing molecules, so even if you have a lot more zinc in your body than cadmium, the cadmium will be able to muscle its way into place with greater ease. Yes, cadmium is a bully.

You'll mostly get cadmium if you live near some sort of industrial setting that involves smelting, battery manufacturing or processing, or other metal-based industries. Or if you smoke cigarettes. Because there aren't enough reasons to not smoke, right?

If you can't move to an entirely new area, at least move upwind of any such industrial areas. You'll easily cut your risk by at least 30% simply by moving upwind instead of downwind of these areas.

Plumber's Bum(mer)

In 2012, the city of Flint, Michigan experienced one of the worst public health disasters in America. Through a series of cost-cutting measures, citizens were exposed to toxic levels of lead, as the toxic metal leached out from the pipes that made up most of their sewers. Children became sick and showed significant damage to their brains. This is truly sad, as the knock-on effects felt down the line will last for a long time while they try to heal themselves from the poison.

For those of you are well-versed in Latin, you know that lead was called *plumbum* back in the good ol' Roman times (and up until the 20th century, to boot). (If you know French or Spanish or other Romance languages, the words are similar.) This is why plumbing is called *plumb*ing — it started out using lead, because the metal is so easy to work with.

The initial benefits of getting water to people in their homes clearly outweighed the costs associated with the lead leaching from the pipes. (Thank you, flushing toilets, baths and showers!) However, we had no idea about the toxic effects of lead at the time.

However, what made lead so great in the first place (the ability to shape it) also became its downfall. Lead pipes would fail relatively quickly. In the meantime, metallurgists were coming up with better materials, such as steel, as well as improved ways to shape metals and alloys. It helps that steel, mainly composed of the abundant metal iron, is much cheaper to source. So the lead pipes were increasingly being replaced with the stronger, less expensive steel, which also had the benefit of being much less toxic.

That said, we all follow the old adage "if it ain't broke, don't fix it". In the case of Flint, the lead pipes were still pushing water to and from homes, so there wasn't a lot of desire to replace the pipes. Couple that with an economy that isn't doing well, and things tend to slide even more. Then things finally broke — people's health. The good news is that, as of December 2017, the US Environmental Protection Agency (EPA) has made replacing lead pipes a priority.

So why does lead have the effect it does on our bodies?

Lead is appropriately called a heavy metal. If you ever get to hold a piece of it, you'll see what I mean. If you're trying to stop radiation, lead is great. It's used all of the time in nuclear facilities for this purpose, as well as to stop x-rays from affecting other parts of your body when you get an x-ray scan.

However, on a chemical level, lead (Pb) has two main forms: Pb^{2+} and Pb^{4+}. The Pb^{2+} binds strongly to the sulphur found in several important molecules in our bodies, much more than most of the elements we need, like zinc. Pb^{4+} will bind to sulphur, but also oxygen-containing molecules. Also, given its size, when it does bind to these sulphur molecules, the shape of the overall complex isn't quite right, so the body can't do what it needs to do with the molecule. Think of it like jamming the wrong key into a lock. You might be able to get the key into the lock, but it won't open it. When you can't open the lock, you can't get to what's inside.

$\sim$

THE TRAGEDY IN FLINT, Michigan, could easily have been prevented, or at least minimised.

As these pipes age, lead is released into the waterways. Without proper maintenance, the lead concentrations increase due to corrosion. (They will degrade completely at some point regardless.)

There are several studies linking the concentration of lead in blood or urine to thyroid issues. If you recall from the chapter on iodine, most of the thyroid issues revolve around the presence of iodine. So far, most studies have simply noted a correlation.

But what's really going on?

Lead binds really, really strongly to iodine.

If you ever want to see a neat chemical reaction, add a solution of lead nitrate (a source of soluble lead) to a solution of potassium iodide (a source of soluble iodine). Both of these solutions go from colourless solutions to instantaneously forming a bright yellow solid. (This is actually what used to be used for yellow paint before scientists realised the issues related to lead paints.) Once a solid is formed, it's really, really hard to break apart those bonds and release the iodine. Which means that iodine that your body needs for proper thyroid function, well, you're going to have to find it somewhere else.

In other words, old pipes (which are pretty much everywhere) + low amounts of iodine (assuming you don't live by the sea and/or eat a lot of seaweed) = potential for thyroid issues.

So what can you do?

First, minimise the amount of lead that you're taking in. For most people, this means filtering your water. This might have to be done within your home, as the pipes feeding it might be old and releasing lead.

Second, ensure that you're getting enough sulphur and selenium (but not too much selenium; see the chapter on selenium). These elements are able to bind lead and help remove it from your body. In fact, both of these are far less soluble than lead iodide (about 10 billion billion times less soluble), which means they're more likely to bind the lead than the iodide is.

Something's Fishy...

Conventional thinking has it that if you get farther away from a source of pollution, you should have less of whatever is causing that pollution in your body. In most cases, this is true. However, there are a few exceptions. One of the most notable ones is mercury.

I've analysed thousands of samples, of just about every species present in the Arctic Ocean and north Atlantic, for mercury. And I can you tell that, while tuna are definitely high in mercury, they don't hold a candle to species like beluga (white whales). Most tuna fall in the single digit parts per million (ppm) range (or 0.0001%) for mercury concentration. Most health agencies worldwide, including the World Health Organisation (WHO) have limits of 1 ppm of mercury for safe consumption, and even then caution against eating much fish that are near these levels. Most of the beluga I analysed, especially their livers, came in at 100-500 ppm. This has some significant impacts for Inuit who rely upon what they can hunt for sustenance.

The Canadian Arctic is pretty far from any large source of mercury: no coal-fired power plants, no volcanoes, no mines and no industry. Industrial sources of mercury tend to spike local and regional concentrations of mercury. Fish in regions of industrial mercury tend to reach up to 1 to 5 ppm of mercury. Yet in the Canadian Arctic, in the absence of these sources, some of the highest mercury levels are observed at the top of the foodweb there, such as in belugas.

Unfortunately for beluga, they're at the mercy of quirks of

nature. It's the unique environmental conditions they find themselves in that drive their high mercury contents.

~

So why is mercury so toxic to our bodies?

We've gone over how cadmium is linked to zinc and can mimic it. But it gets worse...

Guess what's directly below cadmium in the periodic table? Mercury! So not only can cadmium mimic zinc, but so can mercury. And mercury can bind sulphur compounds even more strongly than cadmium can. Yikes!

If you eat a fair amount of seafood, you may have heard warnings about avoiding certain species like tuna and swordfish because of their high mercury contents. This has to do with a process that creates a form of mercury (methyl mercury) that is particularly toxic. Methyl mercury is particularly bad because not only does it bind really strongly to sulphur-containing compounds (especially protein and lots of enzymes needed for life), but it can also pass through the blood-brain barrier due to the methyl group that allows it to sneak through.

The reason why mercury is such a persistent pest is because it binds to the sulphur in your proteins so strongly. You can't just wash it away. You need to get rid of the whole protein, which thankfully, your body does in a process called autophagy (literally, "self-eating"). So if you limit the amount of mercury getting into your body, your body will over time rid itself of the toxic mercury. Two great ways to do this are exercising, which destroys muscle tissues, hence increasing the rate of repair and removal of mercury-containing protein, and by eating fibre and compounds that contain reduced sulphur (see the chapter on sulphur for more details). It doesn't happen overnight, but you can see noticeable differences within two weeks or so.

Assuming you still want to eat fish, if you focus on certain species like salmon, herring and sardines (or any fish that would fit in the palm of your hand), you'll reap the benefits of the protein and omega-3 fats, without going overboard on the mercury or most other organic contaminants.

Now that we've covered some of the toxic metals to avoid, let's look at some organic contaminants.

16

———

ORGANIC CONTAMINANTS AND PLASTICISERS

You can't do everything. You can't go everywhere. We have to pick and choose between good and a little bit better.

— John C. Maxwell

W e're all really good at lying. More specifically, we're really good at underestimating the not-so-good things we do, and at trumpeting up the good things we do.

At this point in time, society has undergone several periods of drug addiction (opium back in the late 19th century, cocaine in the 1980s and the opioid crisis which is on-going today). The scary thing is, unless you live like a hermit hundreds of kilometres away from anybody, you're consuming small amounts of just about every drug known to humans.

Cocaine? Check. Heroin? Check. Marijuana? Check. Prozac? Check. Birth control and Viagra? Yep, you got that right. The list goes on and on...

Now, you might be thinking, I've never even come close to doing heroin! And Viagra? Pfft! I don't need that stuff! (especially so for any female readers). How on Earth am I consuming it?

Simple: you use water.

Anything connected to a municipal water supply (in or out) will be a cumulative pool of everything that has taken place within that system.

For about the past decade, chemists have been finding considerably more drugs of abuse at the inlets of wastewater treatment plants than governmental surveys suggest should be found. The difference is so significant that networks have been developed that measure these compounds in wastewater to get a municipal or regional view of drug consumption. The results are being mapped and are freely available in Europe (http:// www.emcdda.europa.eu/), so you can actually find out the likelihood of drug trafficking in a given region.

So... if we're all getting a little "high", why is this the case? Those poor, old bacteria — the main purifiers of our water systems — simply can't keep up. They're overworked and don't have enough time to do the job they need to do, or they might be missing some key "skills".

What do I mean by this?

We want our water, and we want it now, right? Well, that can make things difficult for our little water-cleaning friends. And the more we use pesticides and medicate ourselves, the harder it is for water treatment plants to keep up...

We pretty much expect to have clean water available to us the moment we open up our taps. Yet there's only so much water that can be pumped through our taps in a given interval. To make sure there isn't a water crisis (like the ones that affected Cape Town in South Africa, or most of California), a lot of the water passes through the treatment plant without being fully cleaned. If you were to see what goes in versus what comes out, you'd be pretty impressed. (I highly recommend visiting your local water treatment plant.) In any case, most of us aren't willing or able to pay the extra costs to beef up the treatment plants, nor are we accepting of not having immediate access to the water (and rightly so!). I live in Canada with an abundance of freshwater and the amount of water the average Canadian uses would probably shock most other people on the planet. I am, however, extremely grateful to live here. (Even if winter can last 6 months or more.)

The other problem is that we're creating new compounds (drugs, pesticides, etc.) every day that don't necessarily break down easily. When you're not only adding more material to process, but also material that's harder to work with, the productivity of a water treatment plant — including the bacteria living within it — drops.

Water Treatment 101

Water treatment plants have two or three levels of water purification, with increasing degrees of sophistication.

The first is called the primary treatment. This is just letting the solids (including *those* solids ranked "second") settle out in what are effectively giant ponds. Often certain chemicals are added to help clump any floating particulate matter to help it settle out. If you're familiar with cats and having to clean out their litter box, then you know your life is a lot easier if you buy the clumping litter. The same idea applies here. Clumping the particulates helps to clarify the water and make it easier on the next step. (Side note: it's common practice to use the solids produced at wastewater treatment plants as fertiliser in agricultural fields. It's not a pleasant mental visual, but it does add necessary nutrients to the soil.)

The next step is the secondary treatment. This is where nature kicks in. In giant retention ponds, bacteria go to town on anything in the water that has passed through the first step. Bacteria do a fantastic job eating up a lot of the stuff that passes through, especially anything biological (regular food for bacteria), and the water that leaves this part of the plant is typically really clean. However, those great bacteria are also forced to contend with anything else that makes its way into the sewers — pharmaceuticals, pesticides, fuel... *Not* their usual food. These things are either harder for bacteria to digest or can be downright toxic to them (like pesticides). However, although some of these chemical compounds can kill off individual bacteria, the bacteria will metabolise these compounds into something easier to digest, which allows other bacteria to degrade these compounds. Providing there's enough time to do so, of course...

Finally, most water treatment plants also have tertiary (third step) treatment. This is chemical or physical treatment of the water to clean it up before it gets into our homes.

Chemical treatment is often by chlorine-based compounds. This is not unlike what goes into swimming pools to keep them nice and clear and algae-free. The chlorine compounds react with compounds present in water and help degrade them. However, this can also produce certain chlorinated compounds that are known to have negative health effects.

As a result, many municipalities have switched to ozone-based treatment. This oxidises most compounds and, for the most part, renders them much more innocuous, either to degrade/metabolise by bacteria present in pipes down the line, or even in our own bodies.

The physical treatment is UV-oxidation. You know how you're always being told to wear sunscreen and cover up when you go out in the summer because of harmful UV rays? Well, the process that causes skin damage is the same one that destroys a lot of chemical compounds, allowing for cleaner water. In fact, most home-based water treatment systems use UV-oxidation for a final clean-up prior to exiting your tap.

However, even with a tertiary system set up for water treatment, there often isn't enough time for all of the chemicals to be removed prior to the water ending up at your home. Put differently, whether you like it or not, you're taking really small doses of whatever else everyone else is taking in your community.

Are we doomed to consume these compounds? Unless we drastically change what we put in our bodies and on our lawns, gardens and fields on a societal scale, then the answer is yes. However, we can reduce our exposure greatly by implementing a few things.

Cut the Crap

First, filtering water through carbon-based filters (such as Brita™) can help. But like the filters on your furnace and in your air intake for your car, these need to be changed regularly. At a certain point, there simply aren't any spots left to absorb the toxins, and they pass through, or new toxins bump out old absorbed toxins. (This is a process known as "breakthrough". Clearly not the kind of "breakthrough" you want.) The more crap the filters take in, the more frequently they need to be changed.

Reverse osmosis (aka "RO") can also help filter out toxins. This works by only allowing really small molecules to pass through a membrane — most toxins get caught in the membrane. Like the carbon-based filters, these systems also need regular maintenance and replacement to ensure your water is getting clean.

There are now several commercial home-based UV-oxidation systems that can be plumbed into your pipes (mainly in the kitchen). More often than not, these are coupled with pre-filters, which really helps increase the efficiency of the UV-oxidation. Toxins can bind to some particles, which helps protect them from degradation, so removing the particles really helps with the process.

Clearly this type of system will cost you more, but it acts like a second water treatment plant, making your water much purer overall.

Too Much of a Good Thing Can Be Bad

One important note: while you want to have pure water entering your body, if the water becomes too pure, that can lead to trouble. Remember that your body is always trying to achieve balance. If the water you take in doesn't have any minerals in it, it will start to take some of the minerals in your body to balance out. If you've eaten way too much salt, this can be a good thing, but generally, it's not.

This is why you don't want to drink distilled water: all of the good salts that were in the water are left behind in the distillation process. Salts like sodium and potassium, responsible for proper nervous function, will be pulled from your body into the depleted water, making your nerves, and by extension your body, respond much more slowly. (In other words, you'll become sluggish, both physically and mentally.) Similarly, distilled water will pull out calcium and magnesium, leading to a host of issues, particularly related to bone health. You also need a certain degree of saltiness in your blood to ensure your heart pumps the blood as it should, so by dropping the saltiness, and hence pressure, you could faint, or worse.

What are some useful ways to ensure that you're getting the right amount of good quality water into your body? You can do some of the following:

- Drink two large glasses of water first thing in the morning. This kickstarts your metabolism and ensures your mind and body are well-hydrated at the start of the day, as it has likely been at least 6 hours since you had any water.

- Try to drink water throughout the day. Remember, water is the vessel of life. All of your bodily functions require it, and it's how your body gets rid of any toxins (chemical or biological). (You know — good ol' number 1 and number 2.) Drink enough and you'll greatly decrease the frequency, duration and amounts of colds and flus you get. There's a double bonus here: if you drink enough water, you're also likely going to use the washroom more frequently, which means getting off your butt and moving around more, which is doubly great for your health!

- If you suspect your water source isn't the cleanest, then invest in a system that will help purify it. Bottled water is often just municipal tap water from an area that isn't overly developed, so you're often just paying for the bottling process and not for any purer water.

All that said, life always has a way of figuring things out. Japanese scientists have recently discovered bacteria that can eat plastic; other bacteria are evolving to be able to break down the various contaminants and drugs we flush down the drain; we (that is, humans) are coming up with new ways to remove these compounds, either by design of the original materials or by better processing methods. Even if we are continually playing catch up.

$\sim$

So where else might you be eating these organic contaminants and plasticisers?

It's no secret that most food is grown with the use of herbicides and pesticides. In general, this has led to an increase in the *efficiency* of how our food is produced, but not necessarily the *quality* of the food produced. This is one of those tricky metrics.

Why? Efficiency is simply measured as completing a task with a set of resources, or in this case, how much food is produced per person or area. It doesn't look at the big picture of *how* it gets done, just that *x* gets done with *y* resources.

It's possible that you grew up on a farm, but increasingly, the odds are that you grew up in an urban area. The odds are even greater that you actually live in an urban area (or at least, not on a farm). I would also guess that you don't work on a farm, nor do you likely grow most of your food. We've swapped out our personal labour for machines and offloaded some of the dirty work (weeding, pest control) to chemicals. This really did increase the amount of food available (while also allowing us to pursue other things that weren't directly related to us getting food). But the quality of our food has suffered.

Obviously, you can eat organic food. You may have noticed that organic food generally costs more than conventional, or non-organic, food. The reason is because it takes more work, and more work leads to higher costs. You might not have the extra money lying around to eat organic, even if you want to. One trick, however, is to buy frozen. It's often just as nutritious as fresh, and because it can be stored for a much longer period, it costs less.

Structured Disruption

As I alluded to above, plastics are a bit more complex. To actually make a plastic, you have to start a chain reaction that usually involves some sort of metal catalyst and usually some form of binder, or "glue", to ensure all of the pellets form together into the desired shape. Quite often the binder will be some form of a phthalate. Phthalates sort of look like a crab (they vary by the size of the "claws"):

Phthalates are the most common compounds leached from plastics — they really do pop up everywhere. The one shown above is known as DEHP (DiEthylHexyl Phthalate), and is by far the most common one, used in things like PVC pipes, shoes, and as a carrier in air fresheners, perfumes, laundry detergent and other personal care products. So unless you never wash, you interact with them several times a day both on and in your body. As a chemist, I see this all the time whenever organic contaminants are analysed — there's always some phthalate popping up with the rest of the contaminants. This mainly comes from leaching of plastic used in the analyses — often from the gloves used to protect the analysts (and sample integrity).

So why is this important? If we look at cell membranes, we can see that there's actually two layers of fats, known as the phospholipid bilayer (plus some protein-based channels). The phospholipids have a part that is happy in water (the round "head" in the diagram, which is the "phospho" part) and another that forms a water-tight membrane (the squiggly lines, which are fatty, or the "lipid" part).

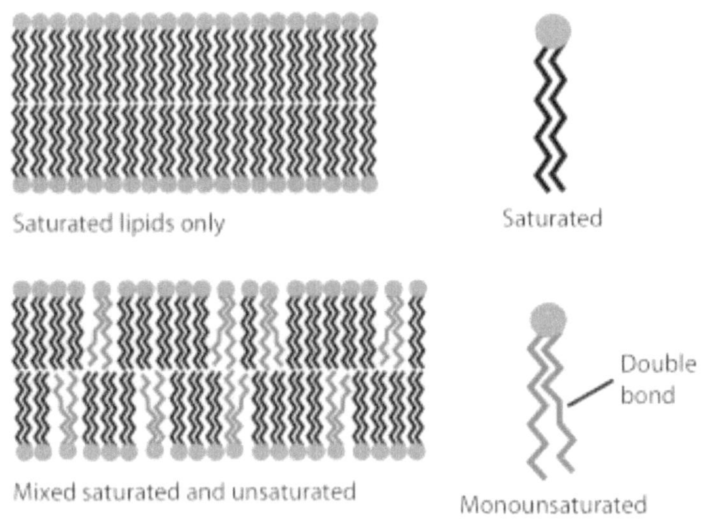

Phthalates, by virtue of their structure, are able to disrupt the cell membrane and create little openings. You want your cells to hold the stuff inside them and stay intact. If you turn them into Swiss cheese, you're gonna run into problems.

A few ways to minimise your exposure to phthalates is to not microwave your food in plastic containers. Heat from the microwave helps to release some of the phthalates, not unlike making the plastic "sweat" a little bit. Once released, the phthalates can then sorb to food. Room temperature or colder is

MUCH less effective at releasing the phthalates. You can also reduce the amount of air fresheners you use. Essential oils, which are all the rage these days, could be contributing to your dose as well. Make sure you know what you're getting into if you decide to use them.

Greased Palms

You've probably seen "BPA-free" plastered on water bottles or other containers. BPA is another plasticiser, or binder. BPA stands for BisPhenol A, so it's kind of like two ("bis") phthalates in one. It has been shown to cause a series of issues with the endocrine system (this produces and regulates your hormones).

However, did you know that BPA is also found on the lining of most aluminium ("tin") cans? It's why the inside of the can feels kind of greasy when you touch it. It also acts a barrier of sorts to the metal leaching into your food, so it's not all bad.

BPA is also present on any thermal paper. You know, any receipts you get printed out when visiting the gas station, grocery store, etc. That's why the paper feels kind of greasy. (Compare with regular paper you would write on, and you'll immediately feel the difference.)

In other words, even if you limit any plastic containers that have BPA in it, you're still getting a dose whenever you handle receipts or metal cans.

Because of the known toxicity of BPA, chemists have come up with similar compounds, such as BPS (bisphenol S). Not surprisingly, these compounds are now being shown to cause similar effects to BPA.

Inputs and Outputs: Detoxifying

The main reason why your body accumulates toxins is because it's taking them in at a faster rate than it can get rid of them. But the great news is that your body is constantly working to get rid of toxins and promote your health. So, by making a few small changes, you can tip the scales in your favour and really help your body get to a lower, healthier level of toxin, and regain a lot of vibrancy.

So how can your body get rid of toxins?

The obvious answer is to not take them in in the first place. The trouble is, that's pretty much impossible in today's world. But you can reduce the amount you take in with the choices you make.

Either way you slice it, you'll need water to wash things away. Your body gets rid of organic compounds like pesticides, pharmaceuticals and plasticisers (like phthalates) by oxidising (metabolising) them. This is mainly done by the liver. Once these compounds are oxidised, they're more water-soluble. This then makes it easier to get rid of them via number 1 or number 2.

Unfortunately, there is no magic wand to eliminate all exposure to organic contaminants. However, we can reduce the risks. This involves WORK.

Grow at least some of your own food. Vertical agriculture (that is, growing food on walls and stacks and not just in large fields) will likely increase in the coming years. This is something that just about anyone can do. All you need is dirt, water and light (preferably natural light, although LEDs are able to do a fair amount). Indoor growing setups (basically trays with grow lamps above) are found just about everywhere these days.

They're great for growing green things like herbs, spinach and other greens. Finally, be okay with the fact that not everything has to smell super-pleasant all the time. Clean is often good enough. Or accept, like most kids do, that a little dirt is just fine.

We've gone deep on the chemical threats to avoid; we'll take a look at radiation and how it affects you in the following chapter.

17

RADIATION

Our world cannot exist without a spectrum that stretches between two extremes to include every variation of light and shade that we sense or experience.

— JULIA WOODMAN

Life is Rad

Let's get a little theatrical, shall we?

I'm willing to bet that at some point in time, you were exposed to William Shakespeare's *Romeo and Juliet*. This masterpiece of star-crossed lovers gives us an important lesson for our health. Let's have a look.

> **Juliet:** *O Romeo, Romeo! Wherefore art thou Romeo?*
> *Deny thy father and refuse thy name; Or if thou*
> *will not, be but sworn my love, And I'll no longer*
> *be a Capulet.*

> **Romeo:** (aside) *Shall I hear more, or shall I speak*
> *at this?*
> **Juliet:** *'Tis but thy name that is my enemy; Thou art*
> *thyself, though not a Montague. What's*
> *Montague? It is nor hand, nor foot, nor arm, nor*
> *face, nor any other part belonging to a man. O,*
> *be some other name! What's in a name? That*
> *which we call a rose by any other name would*
> *smell as sweet. So Romeo would, were he not*
> *Romeo call'd, retain that dear perfection which*
> *he owes without that title.*

Alright, you may be asking, what the heck do Shakespeare's star-crossed lovers have to do with radiation?

Let me ask you a question.

What's the first thing you think of when you hear the word "radiation"? Nuclear weapons? Reactor meltdowns? Cancer? Or in a word, BAD? NASTY? You want nothing to do with it. It's got "Montague" written all over it to your Capulet sensibility.

In many cases, you'd be right about the negative association with radiation. Yet it's interesting that some radiation which is actually quite bad for you is seen as fine, while much more benign radiation is viewed as deadly.

Let's change the wording around a little bit. What if instead of calling it radiation, we simply called it *EM spectrum* (EM stands for electro-magnetic. The "EMF", or Electro-Magnetic Field you hear about falls into this spectrum). Same thing, just different name, or to quote Juliet, "a rose by any other name would smell as sweet". Now, things don't sound nearly as bad, right? Maybe even good?

Radiation comes in a full spectrum, or rainbow (literally). Believe it or not, the simple act of seeing is based on radiation, in this case, the visible spectrum. What's remarkable is that the visible spectrum is a very narrow range (about 400 to 700 nano metres (nm); one nm is one-billionth of a metre). Violet is at the low end (around 400 nm) and red is at the high end (around 700 nm). This is where the terms ultraviolet (UV; radiation from about 100 to 400 nm) and infrared (IR; radiation from about 700 to 10,000 nm) come from:

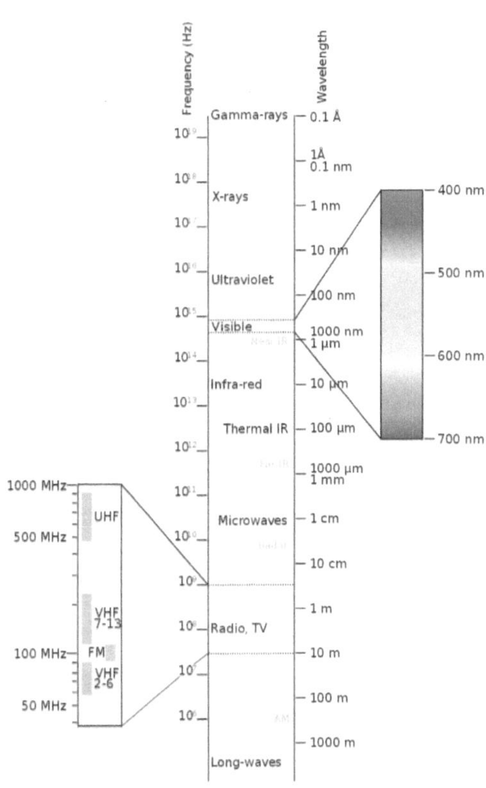

Figure 2: Overview of the Electromagnetic Spectrum
Highlighting the Visible Range

LET'S start at the bottom (energy-wise) and work our way up.

Most of you (I would venture all of you reading this book) have probably never lived a minute of your lives NOT exposed to man-made radio waves. These have been cranking out since they were discovered back in the late 19th century. You know, the AM, the FM. Since they're so low in energy, radio waves are pretty much harmless. (This is not to say it's a good idea to stand directly in front of a radio broadcasting tower.)

Army Popcorn

Moving up a rung on the energy (and frequency) ladder, we get to microwave energy. What's pretty neat about microwave energy is the discovery that led to microwavable popcorn.

One day in 1946, an engineer who was working on improving radar systems had a peanut cluster bar in his pocket while he was working on a magnetron (this emits microwave energy, and is the energy source required in radar detection). Putting his hand in his pocket, he noticed that the peanut cluster bar had completely melted. The important point to note is that unlike chocolate, which *will* melt in your pocket due to the heat released from your body, the sugars holding the peanut cluster bar together require a lot more concentrated energy to heat up and melt. (If you've ever forgotten a chocolate bar in your pocket for any length of time, you've probably come across the sad state of the bar upon opening the package. Sigh...) This melted peanut cluster got him thinking, so he tried an egg (which literally blew up in his face) and then some corn. So, we can thank the US military for microwavable popcorn.

Microwaving food was clearly serendipitous, and just about everyone I know has a microwave oven in their home for this purpose.

How is this actually doing its job, though? Microwave energy works on the polarity of molecules. Polarity is a measure of unevenness in how strongly electrons move and gravitate between atoms in a molecule (atoms like oxygen are highly polar and "hog" electrons, whereas carbon tends to be non-polar). So the more polar elements there are in something, the more they'll absorb microwave energy.

Water (H_2O, or two parts hydrogen to one part oxygen), for example, is really polar. You can easily boil water in the microwave, because it absorbs the microwave energy and then gets hotter. Same thing goes with a lot of food (anything with carbohydrates and protein). They absorb the microwave energy and get hot, or cooked.

Now try doing this with pure fat, like oil, which is barely polar. It will take a lot longer to get hot. Go ahead and try it, and experience this for yourself. Put oil in one container for 45 seconds and feel the temperature. Do the same for water in the same container. The water will be a lot hotter.

While I don't recommend this at home (at all!), I have (in a laboratory) microwaved organic solvents (like what would be found in gasoline) when extracting organic contaminants from soils and various sea creatures (starfish, shrimp, fish, etc.) Unless you add something reasonably polar to the mix (we usually add acetone), the sample won't get hot, and the extraction is basically useless. For the record, lab-grade microwaves are a lot safer to use (and cost a heck of a lot more, too!).

This is all fine and dandy, you might be thinking, but what about liquid egg suddenly becoming solid? What's going on there?

As mentioned earlier, things like protein are great at absorbing microwave energy. There are water-loving and water-hating (hydrophilic and hydrophobic, respectively) parts to proteins. In their native forms, proteins will prefer to be in certain shapes that give them their potency, which is often based on very specific spatial arrangements of the many, many molecular bonds. By absorbing enough microwave energy, these bonds rotate and parts that may have been water-loving before suddenly become water-hating. When parts become water-hating, they start to solidify. (In nerd-speak, they "precipitate" and become "denatured".) This is what happens when your eggs go from being liquid to solid. The bonds aren't breaking apart; they're just re-arranging themselves in space.

As an aside, this is the same process that's happening in the brain of a person with Alzheimer's — proteins are precipitating (solidifying) and lose their function. Not exactly something you want happening in your head (or elsewhere, really).

For this reason, while it's fine to use microwaves to cook your food, don't stand in front of them (or nearby) while they're working. Microwave energy does leak out of the box, and the farther you are from it, the less you'll absorb. A metre or two (3 to 6 feet) makes a huge difference. The moisture in the air absorbs the energy quite well.

Gettin' Hot in Here

Next up is infrared radiation. You and I are infrared radiation sources. In fact, pretty much all of life is. Most of what we know of as heat is infrared (IR).

Remember the old incandescent lightbulbs with the squiggly coiled wire inside? Besides the visual light they gave off, they also released a fair amount of infrared energy. It's why those bulbs in particular got so hot to the touch. (It's also why we need to use a bit more energy to heat our homes in winter, now that we've switched to CFL and LED bulbs.)

Similar to microwave radiation, infrared is mainly involved with molecular motion. However, compared with microwave energy, infrared can also stimulate non-polar (in other words, fatty) molecules. (As you may have noticed, it's possible to have hot oil.) In other words, infrared can stimulate every single molecule in our bodies, including the water that makes up about 70% of our body weight.

IR radiation works by spinning, bending, and stretching molecular bonds. In other words, IR mostly bends, but doesn't break, molecules. (With enough intensity, it will break bonds.) This creates heat — you can think of IR as the exercise of molecules. When exposed to IR radiation, molecules move, dance and shake. Like microwave energy, IR energy also cooks food, and is typically how we cook our food (like in the oven or on the stove or grill).

What's really interesting now, however, is that scientists are realising how important infrared energy is for our health. This is not to say you should go out and literally cook yourself. But you should ensure that you're exposing yourself to some good infrared radiation, like going for a morning or evening walk. Or a nice long, hot bath or sauna. How good do you feel after a nice leisurely walk or soak in the tub? Exactly.

The science here is just in its infancy, but I'm sure we'll start to discover some interesting pathways of how infrared can improve our health.

I Can See Clearly Now

As the name implies, infrared is just beyond the red, or the visible. Visible radiation, at least for humans, is a very tight range of energy — only from about 400 to 700 nano metres. We've evolved to see these colours because they're indicative of the underlying chemistry that helps us live.

All plants require visible light to grow (photosynthesis, or literally, "light-making"). Without plants, there are no insects and animals (including humans). So clearly, kind of a big deal.

These colours help us know when fruits and vegetables are ripe (typically from green to a rainbow of colours). They also warn us of danger (better not lick those brightly coloured frogs).

Some visible radiation, particularly the higher energy blues and violets, are able to break some bonds, particularly those of unsaturated fats and certain pigments (aka antioxidants). This is why many oils, like olive, flax seed, and avocado, are kept in dark glass bottles — they block the light that would transform the unsaturated fats into dangerous peroxides. Unfortunately, this happens really quickly; it only takes a few seconds of blue light to destroy the bonds.

If you've ever looked into someone's window at night and seen the telltale sign of screen time (blue light), know that they're exposing themselves to some relatively harmful radiation. This is why those "blue-blocking" glasses are gaining popularity, and why many electronics companies, such as Apple and Samsung, have a night dimming function to turn down the blue light emitted from screens.

Into the Ultra

After the visible range is UV. We're all familiar with the advice of dermatologists to reduce our sun exposure and use sunscreen. UV is generally highest during the middle of the day, as the sun's rays have the least amount of atmosphere to pass through before reaching us.

UV radiation often has enough energy to break molecular bonds and ionise compounds. Because of this, UV light can create free radicals, which has a series of negative effects in your cells (not all free radicals are bad; your body requires a small amount to do various cellular processes). As mentioned earlier, antioxidants are able to scavenge these free radicals. When you think of your antioxidants, it's a double-whammy: not only do they help to quench any free radicals, but the fruits and veggies that contain antioxidants also have pigments that help absorb the sun's rays in a positive way before they even do any damage. Win-win!

X Marks the Spot

The next step up on the spectrum is x-rays. You may or may not be aware that x-rays are actually quite harmful; they also destroy chemical bonds. X-rays pack a greater punch than UV radiation and easily break molecular bonds, yet many people are more afraid of UV than x-rays. X-rays are more strongly absorbed by heavier elements, which is why bones (calcium, and to a lesser extent, phosphorus) show up so well in x-ray scans. (Calcium has an atomic mass of 40, while your muscle, fat and other cellular material mainly has an atomic mass of 16 or less, and thus appears much darker on x-ray images.) In any case, you should minimise the amount of x-ray scans you get, as they do serious damage to your body.

Going Nuclear

First, a primer on nuclear radiation.

When we think of nuclear radiation, we mostly think of nuclear weapons and the devastation they brought to places like Hiroshima and Nagasaki. As undeniably bad as nuclear weapons are, nuclear processes, which can be harnessed for energy, can be a good thing when done properly. Nuclear processes are indeed extremely energetic and come in four types. So let's get a little Greek and study the alphabet.

Alpha particles. Most people are familiar with uranium and plutonium, the main components in nuclear fuel and nuclear weapons, respectively. There are several other elements involved, but they decay (that is, split apart) mainly by emitting a charged helium nucleus, or alpha particle. (The nucleus is like an atom, but without the negatively charged electrons flying around the core.)

Alpha particles have the curious property of being extremely deadly in short ranges, yet can be stopped by a sheet of paper. It's basically the nuclear version of rock, scissors, paper, where alpha particles are the rock — they smash the scissors to bits, but are blocked by paper. Because alpha-emitting particles are limited in their reach, they are increasingly being used for targeted radiation cancer therapy; specific tumours can be targeted, without a wider dose to the body.

Generally speaking, your exposure risk of alpha-emitting radiation is pretty small unless you work directly with nuclear materials or happen to live in an area with abnormally high uranium or radium content (the other alpha-emitting elements bigger than uranium are man-made). In the case of uranium, this might be certain types of sands (monazite sands, for those who are curious), or radon gas seeping into your basement. Radon is actually the number one source of lung cancer now that smoking is dropping off. That said, there are several measures you can take to clear it out of your house. Your local government should be able to help with this.

Beta radiation. Beta radiation is either an electron (negatively charged) or a positron (positively charged). There are far more isotopes that can produce beta radiation than alpha emitters. The smallest isotope that can produce beta radiation is an isotope of hydrogen, or more specifically, tritium. Beta radiation causes less damage per unit than alpha radiation, but can penetrate farther into the body (typically several millimetres). Some naturally occurring isotopes can be beta emitters; the most important are carbon (carbon-14) and potassium (potassium-40). (The number next to the name refers to the isotope of the element in question.) Other sources of Naturally Occurring Radioactive Material (NORM) are especially prevalent in oil and gas mining operations (the scale buildup on pipes is often high in radioactive strontium and radium).

Seeing as you're not likely to be drinking from pipes loaded with radioactive scale from oil and gas mining operations, let's focus on carbon and potassium. All plants take in radioactive carbon, and in fact, that's how scientists date archaeological artifacts: by knowing how much carbon-14 is left, they can estimate how old something is. (Note: fossil fuels have undergone so much decay that they have no carbon-14 left. This process takes around 25 000 years to complete; compare that to fossil fuels that are many millions of years old, which is why fossil fuels are considered "extinct". The jury is out if these scientists actually had a sense of humour.) However, the overall dose from carbon-14 in plants is quite low and nothing to be too concerned about.

Potassium-40 is another story. Anything that has a fairly high content of potassium (bananas, beans, potatoes) will have a small amount of radioactive potassium (about 0.012%). For a medium-sized banana, this is about 0.1 microsieverts (microSv; this being the measurement unit for radiation dose). A lethal dose is about 3.5 million microSv, so you'd have to eat 35 million bananas, within a day or so, for a lethal dose. It's obvious that you'd die of a lot of other things than radiation poisoning if you were to eat that many bananas so quickly. That said, if you were to consume a lot of bananas on a daily basis (say, at least 5), you would probably set off radiation detectors. This has actually occurred. Transport containers full of bananas have also set off detectors looking for nuclear materials.

Potassium is also very water soluble, so as long as you stay hydrated, you'll be excreting the potassium without any issues. For comparison, a chest CT scan will give you a 7000 microSv dose (or 70 000 bananas' worth), and a three-hour flight would be about 35 microSv (or 350 bananas).

Gamma radiation. Gamma radiation is sort of like a more powerful x-ray. (The power from gamma rays and x-rays overlap a little, but in general, gamma rays are more powerful.) Because gamma radiation are not charged particles, they travel a lot farther than alpha and beta radiation. Gamma radiation is also ionising radiation, meaning that it can break the bonds in molecules (such as DNA). It's actually gamma radiation (normally from cobalt-60) that is used for medical equipment sterilisation, as well as food preservation. (And for those into comics, gamma radiation was how the Incredible Hulk came to be, as unscientific as that may be.)

There's quite a bit of research showing that low doses of gamma radiation have no significant effect on food quality while allowing it to last longer. There was even a study on beef burritos for astronauts on the International Space Station. If you're up in space for six months or more at a time, eating food paste from a tube can get pretty dreary. To boost the morale of the astronauts, scientists at NASA optimised radiation doses that would allow for the beef burritos to last several months without refrigeration, without spoiling or tasting gross. The researchers found that they could indeed extend the life of the burrito to several months with a certain amount of radiation. Beyond a certain amount, however, the burritos turned into goop. And nobody wants to eat burrito goop.

Neutrons. As the name implies, neutrons are neutral particles. Neutrons are able to penetrate a fair distance into materials. The energy from neutrons may damage materials, while a secondary process, called gamma emission, can come from an atom absorbing a neutron, leading to the emission of gamma radiation (i.e., ionising radiation, mentioned above). Beta radiation can also result, depending upon what has absorbed a neutron. Unless you work specifically with nuclear fission or fusion, the odds of you being subject to neutrons in any significant way are pretty much zero.

A Little Bad is Good For You

Okay, I'll fully admit this one's a bit weird, and comes with a pretty big caveat. Recent work is actually showing that *very low* doses of high-energy radiation from UV to gamma rays actually have beneficial effects on the body (a process called hormesis). What scientists think is happening is that there is a small amount of damage from the radiation, but that the body is able to heal and grow, better than if there was no radiation exposure. It's kind of like exercise — you are actually destroying muscle tissue when you exercise, but when the body repairs itself, it comes back stronger and able to do more.

Keep in mind that this is a small window. Higher amounts of radiation are bad for you, and really high amounts will kill you — quickly. You don't want to end up like Alexander Litvinenko, the Russian spy who was poisoned with the radioactive element polonium.

AFTERWORD

There's so much science and information out there these days that it's not only hard to keep up, it can be downright confusing. At the end of the day, while we are making new discoveries from using better tools and new ways of looking at things, a lot of the fundamentals remain the same.

What's great about science is that there are continual improvements. We're now able to detect things at concentrations that were unthinkable not that long ago. In many cases, we can measure parts per trillion (one in a million... of one in a million). This is, frankly, amazing.

Think of the vision test when you go to the optometrist or need to check your vision for your driver's license. We all know that 20/20 vision is great, right? And there are those lines of increasingly smaller letters that only those with really great vision can see... As small as those letters are, imagine being able to read extra fine print at the bottom of that. That's more or less what is possible in many cases. Pretty cool, right? Being able to see ever smaller can only be a good thing.

Well, sort of. Remember what Paracelsus, the father of toxicology, said: the dose makes the poison. Because we know that many things will have negative effects on our health, we often associate *any* amount with toxic effects. And now that we can reliably see things at ever smaller amounts, we become worried about those small amounts.

Going back to the vision test, imagine now that instead of being able to see 20/10 (which is really good, by the way, better than 20/20), you can now see 20/0.00001 (or a million times better). In your everyday life, does this make a difference? Probably not, and in many cases, it might make things worse as you worry and stress about the small things that most people can't see. You'd be too busy avoiding the small amounts of bad stuff to enjoy the large amounts of good stuff.

Does this ring a bell for you or people you know? In some cases, this would be like knowing there's a needle in an extremely large (or several) haystacks and avoiding feeding the hay to the cattle for fear that one would eat the needle and suffer the consequences. Yes, there would likely be negative consequences to the cow that ate the needle, but the odds are extremely small. Most would go hungry and suffer other consequences without that hay.

The other thing to keep in mind is that, provided the dose is low enough, your body is a miracle machine. It will keep you in great health and has the tools necessary to remove small amounts of poisons.

It is my hope that this book was able to explain some of these fundamentals so that you can better understand some of the information that's bombarding you at an accelerating rate. My goal is also to have you become the champion of your own health. After all, you ultimately know what's working for you — and what isn't.

While the overall complexity of life appears to be increasing, there are some simple things that can be done to improve your health:

- Eat a variety of foods. This will likely change by the seasons, especially if your seasons are distinct.
- Eat plants. A lot of them. They don't have to be your entire diet, but I promise you that you will feel your best when you eat lots of them.
- Building on the point above, eat the rainbow, and discover something new to eat. You just might discover your new favourite food. Also, try cooking or preparing foods a little differently. What might have been unpalatable before (boiled beets, anyone?) can become delicious (roasted beets... yum!).
- Make sure you eat a bit of everything, especially all those great F words: Fat, fibre, fruit and "feggies".
- Eat as little processed food as possible. The interwebs is full of great food ideas and recipes.

REFERENCES

This is far from a complete list of all of the scientific literature related to the topics discussed in this book. These references, however, can act as an entry point into further study if you so desire. The information available today is greater than it has ever been, and is obviously showing no signs of slowing down any time soon. The internet is clearly awash is so much information that it's overwhelming.

If you would like to access some of these articles, your best bet is often a university library, or other entity that conducts research with a fair amount of public funding. Several databases exist for focussed searches: Scopus, Web of Science, PubMed, as well as the websites of major scientific publishing firms (Elsevier, American Chemical Society, Wiley, the American Association for the Advancement of Science (they publish Science) and the Nature Publishing Group (they publish Nature and their spinoff journals). The American National Institute of Health (NIH) also publishes a lot of really useful information.

That said, below are some keywords to search for each of the chapters.

Chapter 1: *Uncertainty, error, average, median, standard devia-*

tion. These words will give an idea as to how accurate and precise some of the measurements are. Good studies should state not only what was found in the general population measured (average, median), but how far from that value you can expect to find another value in the same population (in other words, the range of probable values or outcomes). If you see something stating a single value, you should either read a bunch of other studies that give values so that you can get an idea of the range, or take the exact number with a grain of salt.

Chapter 2: *Fat, ketogenic, omega-3, lipid, cholesterol, short-chain fatty acids, medium-chain fatty acids (aka medium-chain triglycerides, or MCT), keto acids, saturated, unsaturated, cardiovascular, neuron, synapse.* These words relate to the kinds of fat available, while the last three relate to heart and brain health. You can also expand your search to include certain symptoms and diseases such as Alzheimer's and dementia.

Chapter 3: *Carbohydrates/carbs, sugar(s), (oligo or poly)saccharide, fructose (and High Fructose Corn Syrup, or HFCS), glucose, diabetes, saturated fat, Fermentable Oligosaccharides, Disaccharides, Monosaccharides And Polyols (FODMAP), irritable bowel syndrome, leaky gut.* There's increasing evidence that overconsumption of simple sugars causes a whole host of negative health effects (diabetes, cardiovascular problems, weight gain, achy joints, etc.). However, carbohydrates have the broadest possible source, which means that you can find them in just about everything. This complexity makes finding any strict links with certain health outcomes (good or bad) difficult.

Chapter 4: *Fibre, gut, microbiome, bacteria, probiotics, probiotics, short-chain fatty acids (SCFA), mind-gut connection, immunity, immune system, intestines, colon, fecal implants, cell wall, leaky gut.* Scientists are increasingly showing that what goes on in the gut is of the biggest importance to our health. The health effects are literally related to the whole body, so there are really no limits to what can be searched for here, although at the time of writing (2018), there's a large focus on mind-gut and immunity-gut links.

Chapter 5: *Protein, amino acids, branched chain amino acids (BCAA), building blocks, muscle, enzymes, collagen, bone density, joints, glutathione, allergies.* Most people will actually exceed the amount of protein they need, especially if they don't exercise vigorously on a regular basis. That said, protein requirements increase as you enter your forties, as your body is not as efficient in building up muscle. Other issues are related to bone density (via collagen) or allergies (such as gluten, peanuts, or shellfish). Look for links to osteoporosis and osteoarthritis in the case of bones.

Chapter 6: *Salt, sodium, potassium, chloride, trace elements, sea salt, iodine/iodised, blood pressure, hydration.* Depending on how much water you drink, how much you exercise, where you live and what you eat, information on salt varies widely, just like the above factors. Relate as much of the information as you can to *your* situation, and act accordingly.

Chapter 7: *Calcium, magnesium, bones, osteoporosis, osteoarthritis, blood pressure, muscle cramps, migraines, depression, mitochondria, energy, dairy, plant-based.* These topics are especially important for women, as they are disproportionately affected by ailments such as osteoporosis, migraines and depression. There are also links to good sleep and muscle cramps in the case of magnesium.

Chapter 8: *Iron, haemoglobin, oxygen, strength, anemia, Reactive Oxygen Species (ROS), free radicals, red blood cells, bioavailable,* *peroxide, iron-sulphur clusters.* Iron bioavailability and the link to free radical/ROS production are the two biggest topics of relevance with iron.

Chapter 9: *Sulphur, cysteine, glutathione, brassicas, cruciferous, sulphur species/compounds, antioxidants, (anti-)cancer, detox(ification), thiol(s), mercaptans, allergies.* Sulphur compounds are generally really good for you. The main thing is to find sources that you enjoy eating. At the same time, allergies to sulphur-containing compounds (think eggs, mustards) can cause issues. Americans spell sulphur with an "f" (sulfur), so just swap out the letters as necessary.

Chapter 10: *Selenium, zinc, copper, antioxidants, selenosis, testosterone, hormones, immune system, detox(ification), growth, brain, supplement.* These elements are often responsible for a host of immune system-related health effects and are often found in deficient amounts. If you have certain health issues related to growth, strength or your immune system, you can look up how these elements interact with them.

Chapter 11: *Iodine, thyroid, TSH, T3, T4, radioactivity, cancer, hypothyroid(ism), autoimmune, Hashimoto's, Graves'.* Big things come in little packages. Your thyroid and iodine might not be large, but they're intricately linked and do a lot for you, especially relating to your immune system.

Chapter 12: *Trace elements, molybdenum, chromium, manganese, antioxidants, hexavalent (chromium), collagen, insulin, metabolism.* There are more elements (such as nickel and cobalt) that also have important health effects, such as cobalt in the case of cobalamin (Vitamin B_{12}), which is responsible for a whole range of things related to metabolism. Detecting what these metals do in the body can be quite difficult, and we're still finding out stuff everyday. Remember, though, that it's the form that these elements are in, and not the total amount, that will have an effect on your body. For this reason, it can be hard to figure exactly what's what with these elements. Keeping an open mind and continually learning is the best option at this point in time.

Chapter 13: *Vitamins, water-soluble, fat-soluble, B-vitamins, supplement, diet, vision, metabolism, immune system, antioxidants, liver, kidneys.* Vitamins do a wide range of things in the body. The important part to remember is that some are water-soluble and go through the kidneys, while others are fat-soluble and go through the liver. The water/fat split is also important, so if you take vitamins in supplement form, make sure you're eating the appropriate foods (such as fat for fat-soluble vitamins).

Chapter 14: *Antioxidants, Reactive Oxygen Species (ROS), free radicals, (poly)phenols, resveratrol, pigments, (asta)xanthins, lycopene, beta-carotene, curcumin, turmeric, epigallocatechin gallate (EGCG).* The antioxidants and pigments all come from plant sources (land plants or marine sources, such as seaweed, spirulina or chlorella). EGCG is one type of polyphenol from tea. While the bulk of research is related to their antioxidant capabilities, there are other effects that are harder to tease out that are currently being studied.

Chapter 15: *Toxic (heavy) metals, arsenic, cadmium, lead, mercury, methyl mercury, tuna, swordfish, rice, bioavailability, corrosion (of pipes), blood-brain barrier, neurological, tremors, Minamata disease, poisoning, detox(ification), chelator/chelation therapy, bioaccumulation, biomagnification, toxicity, respiratory.* There are other toxic elements, but the bulk are covered in the four presented in this chapter. Most of the toxic effects are related to the brain, although they are not limited to just there. Detoxifying from these metals is possible, but just like you didn't get there overnight, getting rid of them won't happen overnight, either.

Chapter 16: *Organic contaminants, plastic/plasticiser, bisphenol A (or S), endocrine disruption, phthalates, cytochrome (detoxifying enzyme group), metabolism, toxicity, hormones, drugs, pharmaceuticals, mimic(ry), volatile organic compounds (VOC), bioaccumulation, biomagnification, persistent organic pollutants (POP), biodegradable, pesticides, herbicides, fungicides, fertility.* There are literally millions of these compounds used widely. As such, there's no real way to escape them. The bulk of the health research is related to endocrine disruption (e.g., hormones) and fertility/viability issues. That said, the solution likely relies on an economic and political solution. Your choices do make a difference.

Chapter 17: *Radioactivity, electromagnetic, nuclear, microwave, infrared (IR), ultraviolet (UV), x-rays, gamma radiation, DNA, single-strand or double-strand break, (free) radicals, hormesis, chemotherapy, radiopharmaceuticals, nuclear medicine, radiation therapy, diagnostics, PET scan, CT scan, risk.* Words matter. We have a collectively negative association with the word radiation, but it's not necessarily so. There are clearly risks involved, but lots of benefits as well. Our modern medical diagnostics rely heavily upon nuclear technology, which has helped save countless lives. I highly recommend an open, yet critical, mind on some of these technologies.

ACKNOWLEDGMENTS

I would like to thank the many teachers — the giants upon whose shoulders I have stood — that I have had over the years. Corneliu Lazar, for getting me hooked on chemistry at such a ripe age. What kid doesn't like to blow things up? Yves Gélinas, for encouraging me to get out of the lab and experience things in nature's lab. Hamed Sanei, you have been a delight and extreme gentleman from day one, not only by taking me under your wing, but in partaking in so many wonderful meals over the years.

Finally, I would like to thank my ever-patient, kind, supportive, smart-as-a-whip and delightfully cheeky wife, Lorrita, for making me pay attention to my health and pointing out the right direction when I was too stubborn to realise the way. It is also her great advice and editing that helped improve this book in many ways.

ABOUT THE AUTHOR

Jesse Carrie, Ph.D., has spent over 20 years studying just about every facet of chemistry from health, to the environment on land and sea, to the fossil fuel, nuclear and power industries. Throughout the years, his analytical toolkit has expanded to cover just about every tool possible, giving him unique insights into how things work.

Jesse has also been a lifelong lover of food, cooking and exploring any food-related lead. His insatiable appetite for learning, growing, and most importantly, eating, has led him to look at how food can be used for optimal health — while being mighty tasty. Who wants to eat gross food, regardless of how healthy it is?

You can read Jesse's food and health-related blog at drjesse-carrie.com. There, you'll find recipes, tips and discussions on the latest science related to food and your health.

9 781999 051808